AVEDA™
RITUALS

Love

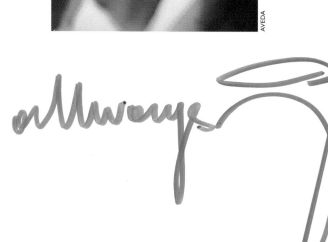

AVEDA

always

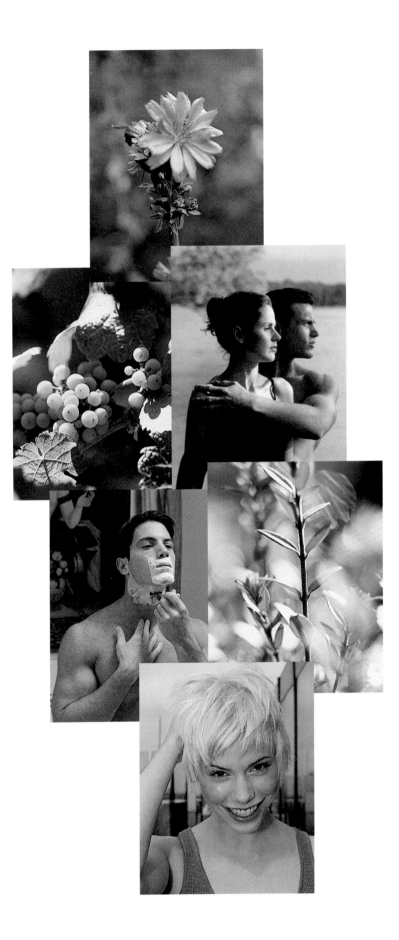

AVEDA™
RITUALS

A Daily Guide to
Natural Health and Beauty

Horst Rechelbacher

AN OWL BOOK

Henry Holt and Company
New York

Henry Holt and Company, LLC
Publishers since 1866
115 West 18th Street
New York, New York 10011

Henry Holt ® is a registered trademark of
Henry Holt and Company, LLC.

Published in Canada by Fitzhenry & Whiteside Ltd.,
195 Allstate Parkway, Markham, Ontario L3R 4T8.

Library of Congress Cataloging-in-Publication Data
Rechelbacher, Horst.
AVEDA rituals: a daily guide to natural health and beauty /
Horst Rechelbacher
p.   cm.
"An owl book."
Includes bibliographical references and index.
ISBN 0-8050-5800-1 (pbk.: alk. paper)
1. Health.   2. Holistic medicine.   3. Beauty, Personal.
4. Mind and body.   I. Title
RA776.5.R426   1999   98-32307
613—dc21   CIP

Henry Holt books are available for special promotions
and premiums. For details contact: *Director, Special Markets.*

First Owl Books Edition 1999

DESIGNED BY LUCY ALBANESE

Printed in the United States of America
All first editions are printed on acid-free paper. ∞

1 3 5 7 9 10 8 6 4 2

Photo credits: Pp. 1, 65, and 201: AVEDA.
Text permissions: Pp. 49–52: excerpt from *A Simple Celebration*, copyright 1997 by Ginna Bell Bragg
and David Simon, M.D., is reprinted by permission of Three Rivers Press; pp. 148–49: excerpt from
The Catalog of Healthy Foods, copyright 1990 by John Tepper Marlin, is reprinted by permission of
The Spieler Agency; pp. 215–19: excerpt from *Healthy Healing: A Guide to Self Healing for Everyone* by
Linda Rector Page, N.D., Ph.D., copyright 1997, is reprinted with permission of Healthy Healing Publications.
Hair styling in "Good Hair Days," pp. 130–41, is by Gina Derry of AVEDA.
Model in "Graceful Motion," pp. 95–107, is DeDee Benrey of the New York Open Center.

This book is not a publication of or by the
AVEDA Corporation. Its contents solely reflect
the opinions of the author.

To my mother, to my teacher,
and to all my mentors
over the years who have brought both
knowledge and clarity to my work

Contents

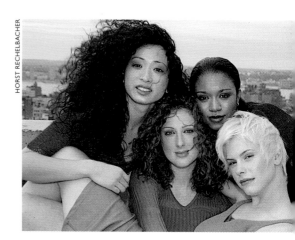

HORST RECHELBACHER

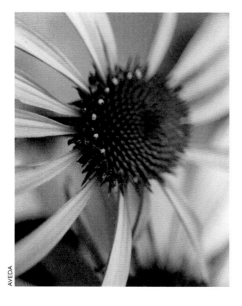

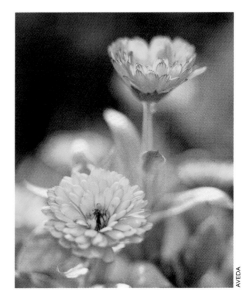

PART THREE · SPECIAL CARE FOR SPECIAL DAYS

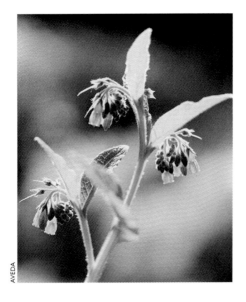

The AVEDA Mission

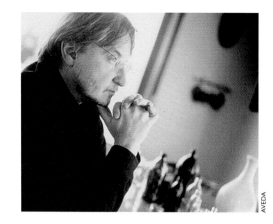

For more than two decades, AVEDA has worked to expand the boundaries of beauty and business, developing extraordinary products made from plants while creating a company with a conscience. AVEDA takes an ethical approach to business: We aim to create products that make intelligent use of the planet's resources; we support the rights of indigenous peoples; we do not conduct animal testing. In our view, these policies make good sense financially, environmentally, and morally. In fact, we believe they are the only sustainable path to the future.

Plants are the starting point for virtually everything we do. They provide essential benefits that support all Earth's life-forms. Through photosynthesis, plants convert sunlight and carbon dioxide into complex chemicals that form the basic ingredients of our food, medicine, aromas, and more. AVEDA's plant-based products draw upon these potent ingredients for their effectiveness. Our research and development team is continually seeking new uses for plant resources and more sophisticated means of manufacture. We go to great lengths to ensure the authenticity, integrity, and quality of our plant ingredients, searching the globe for wild-harvested plants or those grown without the use of petrochemical fertilizers, insecticides, or herbicides.

Petrochemicals are chemicals derived from petroleum. Used as raw materials in the manufacture of many household products, petrochemicals are nonrenewable and can be toxic to people and other living organisms. They pollute our soil, water, air, and bodies. They are widely used because they cost significantly less than pure ingredients extracted from plants. But increased consumption of plant-derived materials would lower their cost, eventually ensuring the ability of the natural environment to sustain itself. For this reason, AVEDA is committed to promoting the use of plant-derived materials.

In the end, issues of environmental and social responsibility will determine the future of our species. At AVEDA, we believe that tomorrow will arrive through the use of renewable resources, sustainable development, and constructive environmental practices. By manufacturing the purest plant products available and using innovative and responsible methods, we are working to set new standards of corporate practice. But the real key to our success, of course, lies in our products. Unmatched in quality and effectiveness, they do what they claim to do. And they do it in such a pleasing manner that you'll want to keep on using them, which is the whole idea.

Acknowledgments

I would like to thank:

Sari Botton, who gave voice to my thoughts

Prakash Purohit, who has been with me at AVEDA for eighteen years

Shivnath Tandof, who has been there through the hard times of AVEDA's development as well

David Hircock, who has shared his wide knowledge of aromatherapy

Teri Gips, whose wisdom on environmental concerns has been a great influence

Joe Gubernick, chief of Research and Development at Estee Lauder, who is helping move AVEDA into the future

Jeanette Wagner, vice chairman of Estee Lauder, for her editorial input

Robby Romero for his friendship and contributions

My personal physicians, Dr. Scott Gerson, Dr. David Simon, and Dr. Donald Hensrud, who are a continuing inspiration to me

Dr. Deepak Chopra, Dr. Candace Pert, Dr. Andrew Weil, Dr. Pamela Peeke, Chief Oren Lyons, all healers of today who are transforming our understanding of health and beauty through plants with their revolutionary work

Dr. Norm Schelly, Dr. Larry Dawson, and Dr. Rudolph Ballantine, who have also been a great help to me

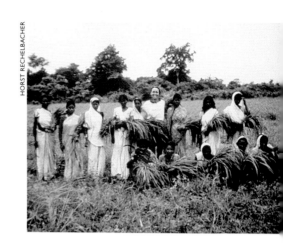

INTRODUCTION

Becoming Connected

You · The Community · The Earth

> *We cannot change the world, but we can definitely transform ourselves.*
> *Self-transformation is essential, and not the reformation of the world.*
> —SWAMI RAMA

WE MUST UNDERSTAND, AS A GLOBAL COMMUNITY, that achieving happiness and wellness is a holistic process. For most of us it is one that requires changes in every part of our lifestyle, changes that include a daily practice of mind-, body-, and spirit-nurturing rituals.

These are not new revelations. The oldest religions in the world and the indigenous peoples who practice them have recognized the power of the mind and spirit for eons. They have practiced simple, holistic, natural wellness rituals for ages as a part of their regular, daily life. Their health and well-being are rooted in rituals and wisdom passed down from one generation to the next. Their answers to psychological and physical ailments are part of their culture and are not the instant, free-floating lose-weight-quick schemes, or the fast remedies for aches, pains, and boredom we often see people reach for today. When most of the Western world turned its attention to this relatively new symptom-relieving modern medicine, a few wise practitioners—doctors such as Andrew Weil, David Simon, and Candace Pert—spent their time and energy rediscovering the ancient knowledge of nature.

My mother was among those who held on to traditional wisdom. She was an herbologist who knew the incredible healing power and intelligence of plants and herbs. Thirty years ago her work inspired me to begin developing herb-based products. After ten years of plant research and study, I founded AVEDA. I envisioned it as an organization devoted to promoting the health and beauty of individuals and the world. I wanted to do what I could through this business to help sustain the plant life that gives us all life.

Not too long ago, health and beauty were thought to be two separate entities that shared little more than an aisle at Woolworth's. The relationship of mind, body, and spirit was virtually ignored, as was the seemingly obvious correlation between the pollution of the Earth and the declining health of its tenants. In the Western world, orthodox Western, or allopathic, medicine was seen as the only respected approach to healing and wellness. This manner of healing was practiced by physicians who did not make any connection between patients' health and their happiness, inner peace, and harmony with the world around them.

Times are slowly changing, though.

Today, there's a return to some of the world's oldest medical practices, global processes that rely heavily on natural plant and herb remedies, including Ayurveda, Asian medicine, herbology, African, and Native American healing traditions, all of which utilize phytochemicals and herbs to balance the body. Now, nearly one-third of all Americans look to the gentler approaches of "holistic," "complementary," or "integrated" medicine to help them cure various ills. In addition, the medical establishment is exhibiting respect for ancient, "alternative" healing practices, including meditation, prayer, yoga, massage, homeopathic medicine, acupuncture, and herbology.

The powerful physiological and psychological effects of aromatherapy are being recognized by many as well. It is not only those in the health fields who see its benefits. A variety of people, including bottom-line pragmatists like casino operators—who have figured out how subliminally to manipulate people into following their noses from twenty-five-cent slot machines to the ones that take only dollars—understand the power that plants and their aromas hold.

It is essential for us to realize that plants are partly healers, and it is in our best interest to protect them. We cannot live without plants, which exhale the oxygen we must inhale in order to live, and which provide vital materials for our food, medicine, and shelter. Plants cannot live in the modern world without our caring responsibly for the soil they grow in and the air that surrounds them. It's an interdependence that needs to be recognized: We need to preserve plants because they are the nutrient carriers from the soil; and we need to heal the soil so that those very plants can thrive. We need to protect all the elements that sustain life—the air, the water, the earth, and the sun.

While we are definitely moving in the right direction toward a more holistic view of our world and health, there's still a long way to go. The pursuit of happiness—not to mention beauty, health, and the ever-elusive fountain of youth—still leads many people to silver-bullet, quick-fix solutions. Aerosol sprays, cigarettes, artificial sweeteners, excessive packaging, and low car-exhaust emission standards are just a few of the easy answers we've turned to that have had an impact on our lives and the Earth. Some of them hurt us directly, and others do indirect harm by injuring the natural world around us. While environmentalism is receiving more media and legislative attention, with recycling becoming mandatory in many parts of the United States, the depletion of ozone becoming an increasingly dire concern, and cleaner air, soil, and water becoming new hot political issues, this is just the beginning. There still isn't enough awareness about the importance of the many steps we can take to be healthier as people and as a global community.

You may wonder why I have decided to touch upon these environmental and activist issues in this health and beauty guide. To me, it makes perfect sense. All of these issues are interconnected with our individual well-being. This book is designed to bring to light that interconnectedness of all things—of health and beauty; of mind, body, and spirit; of our bodies and the larger body we must care for, called Earth. In it, I present an approach to what I call "the business of being," a daily regimen of nurturing rituals that continually promote health, happiness, and beauty both within the microorganizations of our bodies, and the macroorganization of the world.

The book touches on every aspect of life, with rituals for outer and inner cleansing, nutrition, meditation and relaxation, body movement, aromatherapy, massage, skin care, personal beauty, goal setting, time management, and, above all, stress management.

Bear in mind, I use the word "rituals," but you don't have to. I know that for some people that word has negative connotations, associated perhaps with things they've not wanted to do but have been required to do by religions and other people. I encourage you to think of the practices in this book as the options or tools you can choose to incorporate into each day to nurture yourself and improve the quality of your life.

We all have the potential to enhance what we are. We can renew our spirits, energize our organs, refine our body shapes, and heal ourselves and the world around us on a daily basis. However, to do so we must recognize that this is a process that requires skill and tools. It takes the discipline of a daily practice of self-awakening, self-realization, and nurturing of the self and all the things upon which the self depends. It demands our holistic, equal embrace of our minds, our bodies, and our spirits; our insides and our outsides. This is the challenge of creating a truly healthy life.

In these pages I provide a broad menu of daily rituals to help you embrace such a goal, drawing on what I have learned in my own self-exploration over many years. I have studied meditation and yoga in India; participated in Native American ceremonies, worshiped in Buddhist monasteries in Asia, Catholic monasteries in Austria, churches in the American South, in mosques and with shamans all over the world. Through my business ventures and travels, I have met with many religious leaders, including the Dalai Lama and Mother Teresa. I have taken part in global forums at which religious, political, and business leaders, environmentalists, ethnobotanists, anthropologists, and indigenous people have met to discuss ways in which we can help save the environment. The more I have been exposed to various faiths, the more I've realized that all practices of faith lead to peace. You will see that in this book I encourage you to find your own way to peace rather than pushing any one faith or religion. Every path is correct.

In every one of the traditions I've encountered the role of plants is a common element. I have found that essential oils, which are pure essences drawn from plants and then distilled, have been used regularly in prayer and other rituals, as well as for healing. As far back as we can trace, medicine and faith have been highly interconnected in religions around the globe. For example, in medieval times, Catholics in Europe used frankincense—also called olibanum—in their prayers, as well as to help stave off the infection of the plague. They knew what they were doing. As it turns out, frankincense is a great antiseptic! The Moslems use rose attar and ut, from the agar tree, as both antibacterial medicines and prayer facilitators. These are just a few of the examples that show the strong connection between plants, healing, and prayer. This is the ancient foundation of the holistic approach to health, which I will explore and expand upon here in these pages of *AVEDA Rituals*.

I continually study plant essences and aromatherapy, through my work with AVEDA, and nutrition through my work with Intelligent Nutrients, a vitamin supplement company I started in 1995. While some of what I know comes from my own experimentation, a good deal is seated in my more formal training; I have an honorary doctorate degree in Himalayan Ayurvedic medicine from Hadwar University in India. I have written this book to share with you what I have discovered, and continue to discover, on this amazing sensory journey called life.

It is important to note that while many of the simple, gentle practices put forth here are ancient folk traditions, most of their positive effects have been substantiated through scientific research and empirical data. I have been involved in much of this research over the past thirty years and watched the wisdom of folklore become a tangible, effective treatment, again and again.

In the early part of the book, I offer and document the philosophies behind the rituals I present. Later on, I provide a menu of these rituals, which you are invited to consider and incorporate in inventing your own daily regimen. The business of being is a very personal recipe that we all must invent for ourselves, and adjust as we grow. The most important things about your set of rituals are that it nurture you, and that you enjoy it enough to want to practice it daily. It's never too early or too late to start.

AVEDA™
RITUALS

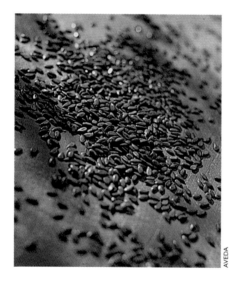

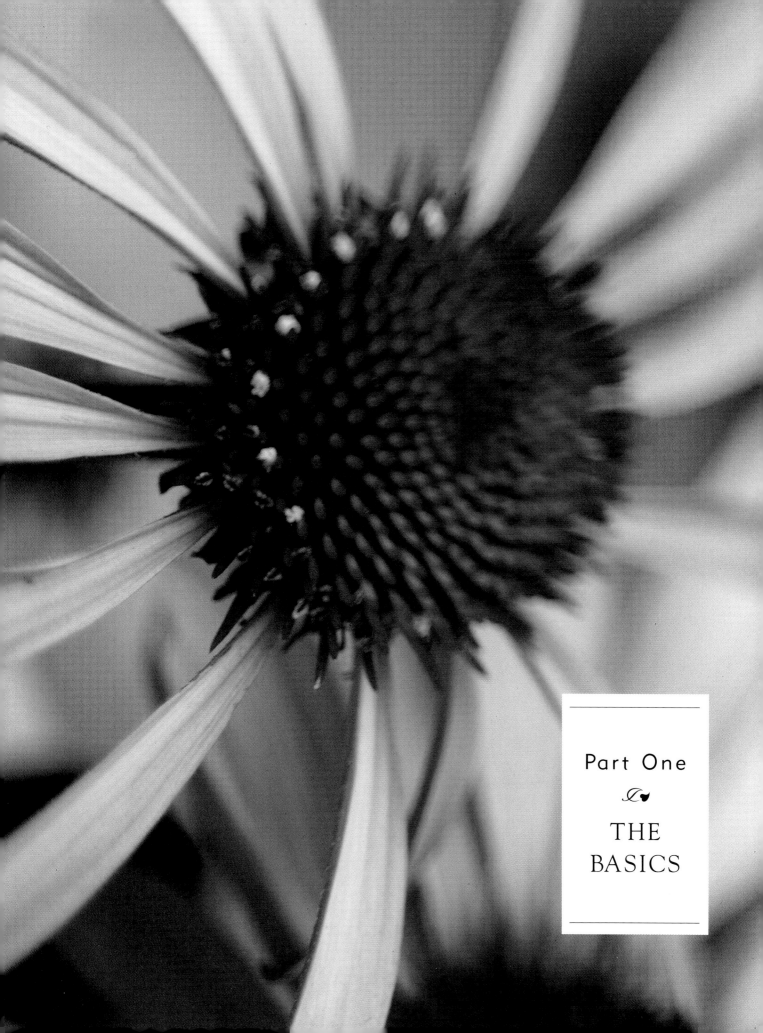

Part One

❧

THE
BASICS

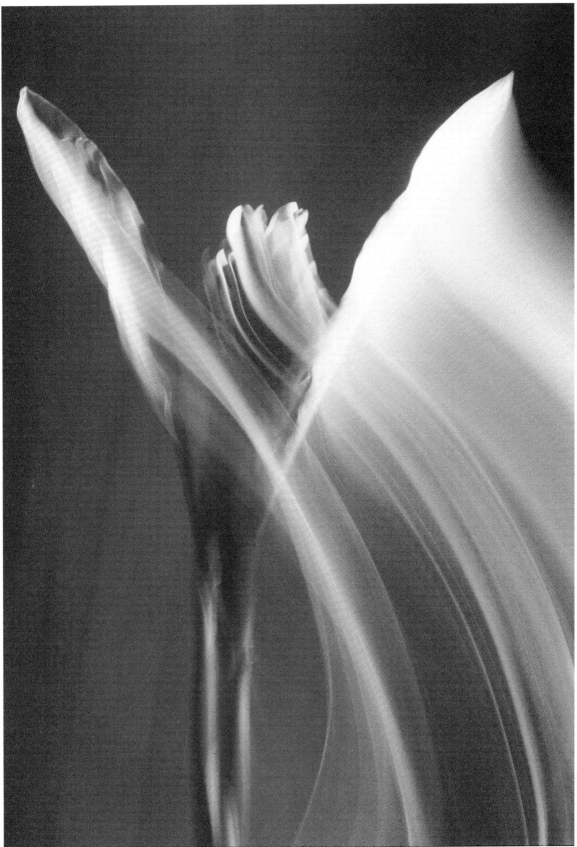

Relativity

If we cannot live for others, life is not worth living.   —MOTHER TERESA

There's only one corner of the universe you can be certain of improving; and that's your own self. So you have to begin there, not outside, not on other people. That comes afterwards, when you have worked on your own corner.

—ALDOUS HUXLEY

DO YOU DRIFT OFF ON A BUSY DAY AND THINK OF an ideal place, one in which you find the time and energy to improve your health, enhance your beauty, and find your personal idea of success and bliss? Who among us hasn't? We all want to feel energetic, content, and youthful, and to have the radiance that comes with such a state. What if I told you all of these goals are within your grasp right here, right now? With the right lifestyle choices, which take into account *every aspect of our lives,* each one of us can create the life we want to lead.

Yet this sort of fulfillment evades most of us. In the modern world, our busy lives and our environment are polluted, both literally and figuratively, with complications and contaminants. We become impatient in our quest for contentment, and lose sight of how we shape ourselves and our environment by the many choices we make each day. That impatience often leads us to dead-end paths—opportunities that provide a temporary lift but no real solutions. Fleeting happiness may seem like a shortcut to genuine bliss, but it is, quite often, a detour away from it.

The forms these detours take are many. Our collective yearning for wellness, harmony, and beauty has given birth to whole industries offering quick fixes, like fad diets, feel-good and slim-down pharmaceuticals, and aisles of fashion choices. However, once the initial thrill of trying something new fails us, we're back where we started, feeling vaguely discontented or further off track. In many cases, we react to this discomfort by immediately searching for yet another easy answer. If only it were as easy as those selling the quick fixes make it seem: Pop a few pills to lose weight and forget your troubles, update your wardrobe, trade in your car for a shiny new one, and live happily ever after, at one with the universe and nature.

It's obviously not that simple. But the key to optimal wellness, inner harmony, and beauty that will allow you to move into the zone of bliss in all aspects of your life is also not as elusive and difficult to attain as it might seem. The path to the fulfillment we seek is a *process*, a way of life, which requires a holistic combination of faith, mindfulness, discipline, and patience. To embrace this *process*, we must put aside the goal-oriented thinking most of us have adopted. We must also return to the basic, infallible intelligence of nature as well as to the time-honored ancient wisdom of wellness and healing that comes to us from the oldest cultures around the world. That means we have to open our minds and our beings to embrace all of life. The information age has driven most of us to live cerebrally. We must remember that there is more to us than thoughts.

This process toward bliss involves nurturing ourselves through all of our senses: feeding ourselves foods that make us feel good; surrounding ourselves with sounds that calm or invigorate us; breathing in pure, plant-derived aromas that smell nice *and* have positive emotional and physiological benefits; creating spaces to live, work, and pray that are pleasing to the eye and welcoming to the spirit; making ourselves beautiful in clothes that feel lovely and are flattering; tending to our bodies with a loving touch and natural plant products.

To enter into this process we must have an understanding and awareness of the relationships among all things. The interdependence between ourselves and the elements—earth, water, air, sun, and space—and our impact on those things that sustain us should influence each decision we make. We must be aware of the complex interconnectedness of mind, body, and spirit; the relationship between our behavior and our five senses; the associations among ourselves and others in our lives; and the inescapable links between the past, present, and future. This is the core of what is called holism, an approach to daily life which recognizes that all things work together or fail together and generally affect one another.

CAUSE AND EFFECT

A successful quest for beauty, health, and happiness cannot be an isolated pursuit we embark upon with our minds set only on ourselves. All things in the universe are associated with one another and engaged in a cause-and-effect relationship. An awareness of that is the foundation of a long-term, nurturing lifestyle. True and lasting beauty emanates from each of our cells when they are balanced nutritionally and stable. The only way we can achieve this deeply radiant state is through healthy eating and centered living. A contented feeling with ourselves and others is key to this way of health—which means those around us must be blissful as well. In order for the world's population to reach this optimal state it must have a supportive environment. This would be a fertile planet complete with rich soil, clean air, and crystalline water. Do you now see the big picture?

There is an internal environment, and an external environment, and the body is constantly relating to each of these. We need to be aware of and manage all of these relationships on a daily basis if we are to fulfill our goal of bliss.

THE INTERNAL DYNAMICS

On the micro level, there is a highly sophisticated set of relationships going on inside our bodies every second of every day that we are alive. When all of those relationships are in check, our body systems function automatically. Even when the relationships among internal organs are less than optimal,

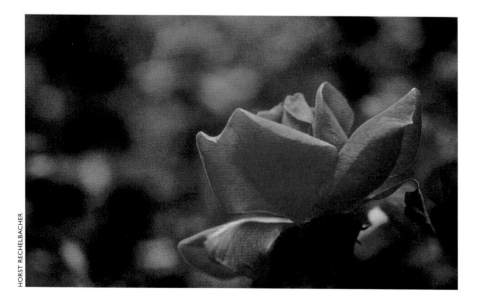

HORST RECHELBACHER

*T*he rose is a symbol of balance, love, and bliss and provides great wound-healing properties.

the body pretty much works on its own and doesn't need direction. When we are in a state of deep sleep, or even just working at our desks, our bodies are functioning on the intelligence of biology, and our individual compositions. Waking or sleeping, we never need to say to our organs, "Okay, it's time to digest food," or "It's time to circulate blood," or "Time to lubricate the skin with secretions from the oil glands." That is all done automatically with no conscious direction from us.

But there is another dimension to this relationship between ourselves and our bodies through which we *can* and *do* have an effect on the quality and efficiency of these functions. Although our bodies are on automatic pilot and will perform for us regardless of our lifestyle choices, there is no question that they will serve us better when they are nurtured. To understand each of our individual body's needs, we can learn about its particular inclinations through the tradition of Ayurveda. The wisdom of Ayurveda helps us to design a complementary diet and way of exercise for our particular body type. In the next chapter, I'll discuss the three *doshas*, or body/personality types, put forth in the Ayurvedic tradition, and how you can use this information to tailor a lifestyle specifically suited to your body's needs.

When we choose to surround our bodies with clean air, and feed them with nourishing, organic food, purified water, and a healthy dose of sun, we help them to stay healthy and balanced. When we pay attention to their particular compositions, treat them internally and externally to the miraculous benefits of pure plant and flower essences, our bodies respond positively for the long term. We promote wellness, longevity, radiance, and bliss when we follow simple, nurturing practices, including:

- yoga
- aerobic exercise
- mediation
- making positive contributions to our world
- aromatherapy with pure plant essences
- herbology
- inner and outer cleansing
- eating intelligently
- self-massage
- partner and family massage
- goal setting
- conferring regularly with doctors, trainers, and other "coaches"
- being aware of and controlling our breath
- listening to our bodies

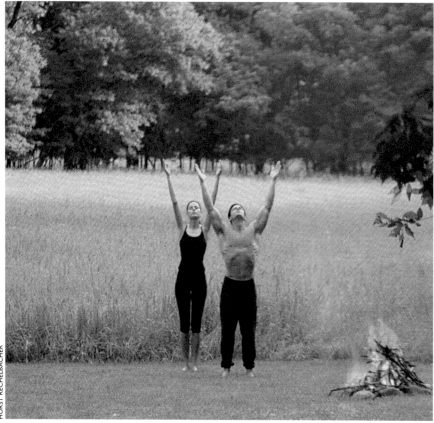

HORST RECHELBACHER

Yoga's breathing and movement connect our mind and body; practiced outdoors it can link us to the natural world around us.

Generally, when we avoid things that cause stress, or "dis-ease," we avoid illness or disease. Sometimes it is difficult to distinguish unnecessary disease from the natural stress, or pain, that is part of our personal development. The latter is necessary, and we must work through it to achieve bliss, unlike the needless stress that results when we take shortcuts, or temporary happiness routes. As you go through the book and focus more on yourself and your goals, that distinction will become easier to make.

Yet another layer of relationships in our bodies involves the connection between our physiological and psychological well-being. Ancient medicinal traditions have always addressed this connection and suggested health practices for enhancing it that allow us to enter the zone of bliss. For example, yoga, one of the most ancient practices, gets its name from the Sanskrit word for the union of the mind and body. The chakra system, from Ayurvedic medicine, takes into account the human urges and emotions, and our bodies' physiological energy/information centers where they develop. It is helpful to incorporate one of these practices into your daily regimen in order to facilitate the union of your body's various internal, interconnected systems.

THE CHOICE IS YOURS

We can make changes in our own lives and behaviors that enhance our natural balance and combat dis-ease; these changes include:

▸ spending more time in nature

▸ driving our cars less and car pooling more

▸ buying quality durable goods that will last longer and thereby reduce the strains of manufacturing and waste on the environment

▸ recycling

▸ supporting organic farming because it promotes clean soil, air, and water and better nutrition

▸ avoiding products and services from companies that pollute

▸ refusing to buy beauty products in which petro-chemicals are the main ingredients

▸ engaging in business practices that are positive and help to sustain natural resources

▸ looking for the good in everything

Today, scientists like Dr. Candace Pert are able to document scientifically the effects of emotions on the health of cells. In her book *The Molecules of Emotion* (Scribner, 1997), Dr. Pert gives scientific language to the phenomenon of healing our bodies by first healing our minds and our souls, which monks and yogis have been doing for millennia. We produce and release neuropeptides—immune system building blocks—when we feel nurtured. As a result, even those of us with depleted immune systems, such as AIDS or cancer patients, can benefit. I recommend reading this book, written by one of the most brilliant scientists I have ever met.

THE EXTERNAL DYNAMICS

Outside our own bodies, on the macro level, we have an ongoing relationship with the universe. The world around us encompasses both the grand universe at large and our own personal orbits of environment and forces within it. Sometimes the links we have to our outer world are subtle. We aren't always aware of the effect our surroundings are having on us, or the effects we're having on our surroundings. For example, when we are in the country, the trees, silent as they are, have a tremendous influence on us. When we are surrounded by them, we are affected in a profound and positive way. These trees cleanse our air. They take the carbon dioxide that we exhale and turn it into oxygen for us to inhale. This simple interaction is the basis for our general health. Each breath we take in of clean, oxygen-filled air is a healthy one.

In contrast, when we transport ourselves to the city, suddenly we are surrounded by man-made electromagnetic vibrations, air and noise pollution, as well as toxins and diseases of all kinds. In these busy places there is also a change in the rhythm of the electromagnetic field around us, which changes the rhythm within us. The intensity of those rhythms can be toxic; anything that puts stress on our beings *is*. All these things affect the body in a very profound way. They put a strain on the liver and the kidneys. They disturb our sleep and our digestion. They put stress on our skin. My skin rarely breaks out when I'm at home in Wisconsin, but as soon as I go to New York City, I know I can expect one or two breakouts. All of these subtle and not so subtle changes also have an impact on how we think and how we function.

When we are aware of how elements of the outer world interact with us, we can make choices that adjust and improve our relationships with the world as a whole. We can make choices that adjust and improve our relationships on the macro level.

ASK NOT WHAT YOUR PLANET CAN DO FOR YOU . . .

This brings us to the next logical relationship in our lives: that between our inner microcosmos and our outer macrocosmos. When we consider only the microcosmos of the self, and listen only to the urges that occur there—such as the desires for food, sex, sleep, and entertainment—we often forget about how each of the choices we make influences the world around us. Lately, so many of us have forgotten how our actions can and often do interfere with the collective urge for the preservation of life that we have begun to put our surroundings and the life they hold in danger. If we think only about filling our bellies and don't consider whether our food is treated with pesticides that harm the environment, then we may not have a healthy environment for much longer. And it won't matter, because as part of the life that this Earth sustains, we as people are endangered ourselves. In the end, if we don't make a change, we won't be here anymore, either.

It is important to be aware that we each come equipped with two natural urges: to preserve the self, and to preserve everything to which the self is related. These must not be separated. In order to sustain the life of the individual, we must sustain the larger body, the Earth. This is a very basic, but often overlooked, principle of biology called interdependency.

I have always been inspired by the words of President John F. Kennedy, even when I was very young and lived in Europe. I think one of the most profound things he said was, "Ask not what your country can do for you; ask rather what you can do for your country." I talked about that once in a lecture I gave that was meant to motivate people to participate in organizations. In my lecture I said whoever wrote that speech of Kennedy's must have been a biologist to understand that concept of interdependency and highlight its important message of feeding those things that sustain you. At the end of the evening, a woman came up to me and said, "You were right. My dad wrote that speech, and he was a biologist." She was surprised by my observation. I have always felt everyone should have as firm a grasp on interdependency as biologists do. Unfortunately, few do. If this were not the case, we'd surely have a greater movement toward preservation of all that surrounds us, and I would not have been able to draw the conclusion about

THE BIG AND THE SMALL OF IT

What are the microcosmos and the macrocosmos? Those are really relative terms. They are meant to convey a relationship and can be different things in different instances. For example:

- When we're talking about our bodies, it is our physical selves that are the macrocosmos, while our individual cells are the microcosmos.

- When we're talking about the world at large, our bodies are the microcosmos and the Earth is the macrocosmos—the little body and the big body.

- On an even grander scale, when we talk about the universe, the earth is the microcosmos, and everything else out there is part of the macrocosmos.

I use these words to refer to the relationships between these things, and as a reminder that large things always rely on the small things from which they are constructed. When the larger entities are suffering, all the smaller entities within them suffer, too.

who wrote Kennedy's speech so easily. The message is, you have to constantly give to the system without asking for anything to come back. Mother Teresa also focused on this when she said: "If we cannot live for others, life is not worth living."

But biologists and spiritual leaders are not the only people who have seen the importance and benefit of acknowledging and honoring interdependency. It's also a successful entrepreneurial concept that helps to build a productive organization. Give to your employees, and they will work to sustain an organization that gives back to you. If you approach your life that way, in what I call the business of being, then this dynamic can work for you on an individual level, too. Give to the people and things that sustain you; nurture and support all that surrounds you and relates to you, and you will be nurtured and supported in return.

HEALTH + BEAUTY = ENVIRONMENTALISM + ACTIVISM

One important macro way to begin practicing interdependency in daily life is to become an environmentalist. In these times, we cannot afford *not* to be environmentalists and activists. We can't separate ourselves from the environment anymore because we rely on it so strongly, especially since our population keeps growing. If we keep depleting and polluting the environment, we end up destroying our own systems. To reinstate a healthy balance we all must become activists by supporting only those activities and companies that put back into the environment as much as they take out. That way they don't break the cycle of sustainability.

Modern times have influenced how we interact with the elements—the earth, the air, the sun, water, and ether, described in Ayurveda as earth, wind, fire, water, and space. In the past two hundred years, we have inflicted more destruction on ourselves and the world around us than ever before in documented history. Just the additional hardship on the Earth and its resources caused by population growth is staggering. In the seventeenth century, there were only about 4 million people living in what is now the United States. There are now about 250 million inhabitants on the same piece of land. Because there are so many of us, each of us now has to be that much more careful about our actions and our consideration of how they affect the world around us.

To get on the right track again, we must start at a very basic level. The earth itself, the soil, needs to be renurtured so that plants can be sustained. What plants give off during photosynthesis is what we inhale, so plants are, by nature, our life support. Plants also feed us and the animals around us.

Plants are chemical engineers, too—they are the source of natural medicines. They carry thousands of years' worth of information within their biologic structures. Unfortunately, some 90 percent or so of the plant species that exist on this planet have not been studied for their healing properties or natural elements, which is a shame. In the past two hundred years, we have evolved into an intellectual society that has found it less expensive and more efficient, in some ways, to reproduce nature's effects artificially, through chemistry. Synthetic alchemy allows us to produce fragrances and substances that carry the right scents or chemical compounds to please our senses or address our symptoms. But these man-made substances carry none of the other complex medicinal or aromatherapeutic information of the original plants and flowers they're mimicking.

Another big dilemma that we face as a planet is that we are cutting down many of the forests for industry and for real estate in a practice known as clear-cutting. When we lose forests, we lose the intelligence and natural faculties of plants in huge numbers. When plants and trees disappear, the soil becomes depleted of nutrients. This cycle of destruction and depletion of natural resources will soon catch up with us and become irreversible if we are not careful.

I will say it again—our potential quality of life begins and ends with the quality of the soil. You reap what you sow. We need to start with healthy, rich soil if we want to have healthy lives. As consumers, the most powerful and productive way for us to promote healthy soil is to support organic farming. By avoiding pesticides and using purified water, organic farmers produce the most nutrient-rich fruits and vegetables that, in turn, enrich the soil so that future crops can be fortified as well. As a result, the animals and humans who eat the organic food create less harmful waste, which has less of a toxic effect on the water, and later the soil, through which it passes. If we advocate organic farming—en masse—we will set in motion a cleansing cycle that could eventually repair most of the damage we have done to this planet. There is hope!

AWAKENING

In order for the world's population to bring about a nurturing, environmentally aware and active new future, each one of us as individuals must be alert and awake to the holistic nature of our existence. This is really the foremost, ongoing challenge we all must embrace as human beings. This is the path to the balance we must reinstate in our inner and outer worlds.

You may think that just because you're reading right now, or because you have your eyes open, you are awake. On a certain level, you are. But are you really mentally, consciously awake, open to all the realities of your life? Are you aware of the pace of your own breath, and of the fragrances and sounds

---

LABEL AWARENESS

Nonsustainable petrochemical ingredients used in cosmetics:

Propylene Glycol
synthetic solvent and conditioner

Butylated Hydroxyaninsole, Butylated Hydroxytoluene (BHA/BHT)
synthetic antioxidant

Carbomers
synthetic stabilizers

Isobutane, Propane
hydrocarbon propellants

Musk Xylol, Ketone
artificial fragrance

ANIMAL-BASED INGREDIENTS COMMONLY USED IN COSMETICS

BLOOD
  moisturizing creams

LIVER
  nutritional supplement

BONES
  desserts, yogurts, candies, cigarette papers, stamp adhesive, bone china, capsules for pharmaceuticals

HIDE
  cosmetic treatments, wound balm

INTESTINES
  soaps, creams, cosmetics

FAT
  soaps, lipsticks

that surround you? Do you stop to actually taste your food as you're eating it? Are you aware of your goals—for the day, for the week, for the year, for your lifetime—and how this moment affects your achievement of them? Are you aware of how they affect the world around you?

In modern life, it is frighteningly common for people to go through their days asleep, doing everything they can to avoid the slower, more tuned-in processes that yield growth and, ultimately, contentment. There are so many impulses that tempt us to check out mentally, emotionally, and spiritually from our own experiences, especially when we run out of patience for the gradual process of personal development. Distraction is available everywhere in our midst—on the television, on the Internet, and at the shopping mall. This constant pull on our attention dulls our senses, which are vital to our experiences as tools for our development.

When we use these distractions to suppress emotions, such as anger, sadness, and jealousy, those feelings may manifest themselves in physical ailments in a predictable way. The chakra system, which comes out of the Ayurvedic tradition of medicine, offers a very clear understanding of the way in which emotions affect specific organs and their functions. Refer to the chakra section in Chapter 4 for a comprehensive chart on these vibrational zones and their relationships to our minds and bodies.

To avoid this dis-ease and not spread it into the world around us, we must work in life to pay attention, to adopt a conscious, eyes-open-wide approach, which the Buddhists refer to as *mindfulness*. It takes discipline and a new focus in order to do this, but the rewards are many. For example, we can adjust and improve many of the subliminal relationships we carry on within our internal and external worlds when we bring them to the conscious level. Certainly these interactions can continue on, straight ahead, without our mindfulness. But real growth and improvements to our quality of life as individuals and a global community depend upon our willingness to be awake in our lives and to make positive, nurturing choices.

The quick-fix solutions many people seek are often the result of an unwillingness to be present and conscious in life. Many will do anything to escape the growing pains that are a vital part of human experience, and which are, in fact, great opportunities for us. Experiencing emotional pain is a natural part of life. It is a teacher, and an opportunity that can lead us toward contentment. When we look at it this way, we can gain a great deal from the suffering we will inevitably encounter in our lives. Avoiding pain only causes it to resurface and/or accumulate. We have a tendency to forget this in our society of instant gratification and relief. The way we treat illness is a perfect example of this system. In Western medicine, when we treat only symptoms—usually some form of pain—we often only postpone dealing with that pain, which will reappear later. Or we cause new pain, in the form of side effects from the "cure." This approach to healing deals only with effect, and not with cause, and so the cause of pain goes unchecked but suppressed, while the effect of pain is merely rerouted. When we look closely, we see there is no cure of dis-ease or disease without finding the cause of the disease and addressing it. The same goes when we look to attain personal growth and fulfillment. Often there are issues that require our attention and nurturing if we are to move beyond our current limitations, growing into the complete person we are capable of being. Many times this growth is uncomfortable on one level or another. We must work through that stage, however, to reach a new pain-free level of being.

We see the benefits and progress of such a movement through stages of pain to bliss in yoga practice. In working through the pain of a particular position, you breathe through the difficulty and gradually resolve it. After a few times, when you go into that pose again, you will not feel pain where you felt it before. You will have moved into a deeper expression of it and, in so doing, advanced to a new level. We move through emotional stages in a similar way.

For many of us, just dealing with reality of any kind—whether it's our job, our relationships, our weight, our financial situation—is a source of emotional pain. Our first inclination is toward all sorts of avoidance of it. To escape the emotional pain associated with what's happening in the moment at hand, we dwell in the past or project the future. We harp on what *could have been* done differently, or dream about how we're *going to be* better (workers, dieters, savers) tomorrow . . . and tomorrow, and tomorrow. Though we all follow it, we all know how ineffective that plan can be.

Being present in the present can be a challenge, but a most worthwhile one. When we pay attention to the here and now, we are in a healthy relationship with our surroundings and can draw much more from them. The move into the present can start very simply with subtle changes in our awareness of ourselves and our surroundings and constantly dealing with suppressed emotions. We need to continuously analyze and observe ourselves, to live in a state of mindfulness. That which bothers us can only be healed when we are honest in acknowledging that it exists. Through mindfulness, we can figure out the causes of emotional pain, let go of the bad habits that cause it, and adopt new habits that bring about more positive feelings.

To start on this path of self-awareness, you can begin on a very micro level, with an awareness of the most basic, necessary human function:

breath. In many ancient medical traditions, breath is described as the grounding device. In every tradition I have studied, from the rain forest medicine men, to the shamans in the African tradition, the yogis in the Himalayas, and to the medicine men in the Native American tradition, breath plays a key role. These traditional medical practitioners know from wisdom passed down for thousands of years that one of the best ways to become conscious of self is through awareness and control of breath. We in the West are just now coming to see and use this knowledge in our lives.

The ancients of many cultures knew what we are now discovering—that there is a vast ocean of information surrounding us, inside and out, that's similar to all the information on the Internet. It flows through us and around us. Our breath can be like a computer program that can actually help us plug into that sea of information. When we ground ourselves through the breath and move into a low vibrational state, which is close to what is called the alpha state, then we can blend ourselves into nature's information system, and even the cosmic information system. By grounding ourselves into a very focused state, we are able to become much more aware of, and balanced with, the vibrational levels of the other things around us, and to make salient decisions about the things we do and don't want to participate in. Taking an aware breath is like playing an instrument that's in tune with the rest of the orchestra. Playing in tune, being in balance with the vibrations around us, gives us a feeling of joyful harmony, rather than discord.

Being aware of breath, and controlling breath by doing certain breathing exercises, are crucial practices for us as we look to improve the wellness of our mind, body, and spirit. It is the first building block to the business of being, which allows us to become more clearly aware of our senses. When we are aware of our senses we help our brain manufacture neuropeptides, the immune system building blocks that help our bodies to stay healthy and strong through feelings of nurturance. Slow down the processes of life and become an observer of yourself on a full-time basis. You will be giving yourself the best medicine of all: a balanced system of self.

We can uses our senses to affect our thoughts and, ultimately, our outward actions as well. Our brains are like intricate computers that get their input from our senses. The result is what we know to be sensory perception. The limbic system, a storehouse of memory in the brain, is a very efficient data bank that stores all sensory experiences. It memorizes our actions and reactions. Everything we have ever smelled, tasted, seen, felt, or heard in our lives since conception is remembered and referenced there.

So, when you go through a sensory experience, your brain goes on a search through its memory bank to tell you whether you love it or you hate it, whether this is a nurturing or a painful experience. Many of us go through life accepting the response that our brain retrieves and provides. We automatically respond to that by avoiding certain pain-causing situations in the future and moving toward pleasure-generating ones. We don't process these action responses or examine them. Many of us are not aware of what drives our behavior and therefore are not healing or advancing our emotional state.

Opening our eyes to the intricate function of our minds and bodies can lead us to the growth and development I have been discussing. We can manage these data banks ourselves, so that the information we input through our daily rituals can have positive results. We can change the existing data, so that something that our brain perceives as nurturing but really is not, such as nicotine, can be newly understood as a negative influence. In the next chapter, I'll talk about using aromatherapy to feed the brain specific messages that evoke certain feelings and inspire particular behaviors.

We must also become aware of which experiences arouse fear or stress in us, and what physiological changes arise from that, so that we can change both our perception of them and our physical reaction to them. In doing so, we are able to reduce the subtle trauma our systems receive and fend off dis-ease. For, at the moment in which we identify an experience that is nonnurturing, inspiring fear, hate, or jealousy, our bodies' natural reaction is to move out of the zone of bliss. Our body chemistry changes, our heart rate increases, brain waves become high-frequency, blood vessels contract, body temperature drops, and muscle tension increases. Our body is in a state of "red alert," out of balance and being drained of its energy. In this state, the body is actually manufacturing and promoting toxicity. That directly affects our organs. The greater number of these negative reactions our mind perceives, the weaker our whole physical system gets.

Fear is the largest blocker of all systems and a huge cause of stress, emotional and physical. The most important things that I have learned in my studies of health and wellness around the world have been about creating practices and treatments—mental and physical—that conquer fear in the mind. Understanding what causes fear can help us change our emotional state and turn a crisis into an opportunity. Each of us as an individual needs to invent a ritual or a set of rituals to be practiced that reduces our fear and increases our bliss. We must work to develop a practical, healthy management of our thoughts. These practices are meant make time and space for your thoughts and allow you to create your own healthy thinking. We'll talk more about finding sanctuary and creating rituals for healthy thinking in the next chapter.

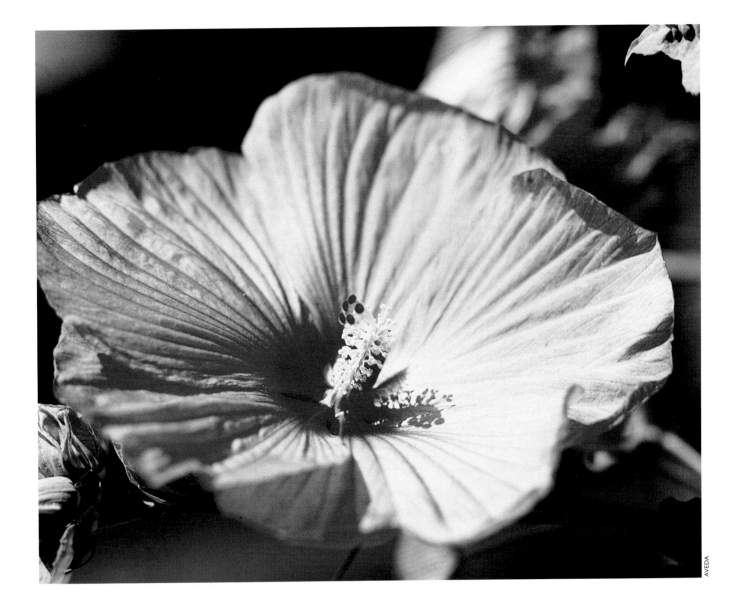

2

The ABC's of TLC

A Nurturing, Conscious Approach to Self-Health Care

You are the architect of your life and you decide your destiny.

—SWAMI RAMA

D O YOU REALLY BELIEVE THAT YOU CAN BE A HAPPIER, healthier, more successful and beautiful you? Think about this question for a moment. It's a very important one. Before you can achieve any of these improved states of being, you must believe that you *can* achieve them, and you must have faith in the power of your own will and choice making to get you there. Only then can you submit to a new life process and reap the benefits.

Once we accept that better living is a matter of choice, a whole world of self-enhancing possibilities opens up. Let's take a look at the variety of lifestyles and nurturing practices we can choose to incorporate into our daily rituals. Here I'll introduce you to them; later in the book, I'll elaborate specifically on how you can put these concepts into practice.

While I can suggest a path, each of us must navigate our own personal route to optimal health and well-being. You must decide where you want to go, how to get there, and what tools you'll need. In order to determine my course and stay on it, I have found planning and mirroring to be invaluable. As I go along, I stop and reflect on my short- and long-term goals, see how

NUTURING RITUALS

▶ establishing a well-rounded network of trustworthy coaches, mentors, or personal trainers, who can help you map out and stick to your path

▶ meditating regularly

▶ becoming aware of and controlling your breathing

▶ practicing your faith

▶ soothing and exploring your mind with the real plant and flower essences of aroma-therapy, and through humor and moments of sanctuary

▶ using plant-based, non-petrochemical cleansers (for your body and home), moisturizers, sunscreens, hair-care products, and makeup

▶ introducing daily self-massage, as well as massages by and for a partner, into your routine

▶ incorporating a combination of relaxing and invigorating body movements, such as yoga, tai chi, and aerobic exercise, to work through stress and maintain optimal body condition and function

▶ eating only organic foods

▶ balancing the chemistry of your diet intelligently, with good amounts of protein and essential fatty acids, and a modest amount of carbohydrates

▶ tailoring daily diet and eating habits to your specific needs, using the wisdom of the ancient indigenous traditions and the latest scientific discoveries about food chemistry as it relates to body chemistry and blood type

my current choices, rituals, and actions are leading me to them, and make adjustments as needed. I will share how I've used these tools and suggest ways you can tailor them to suit your personal needs.

MIND OVER MATTER

What are your beliefs concerning the state of your own well-being? It's a good idea to consider them before adopting a new set of rituals. Have you always recognized your responsibility and power in shaping your life and your outcomes? Are you aware of your relationship to your own happiness, health, success, and beauty? Or have you considered yourself a victim of circumstances, always fighting uphill battles and following the rules of every game to no avail? Have you blamed your lack of satisfaction on people and things outside yourself? Your parents? Your significant other? Your genes? Your job? God or the Devil?

When we are invested in believing that outside factors and other people rule our destiny, it is difficult to expect that making new choices for change will have any positive effect on our lives. After all, in this mode the thinking goes that the last set of choices we made didn't work, presumably because of outside obstacles, and so, even if we give something new, like the AVEDA rituals, a whirl, they probably won't work either. All those people and circumstances are still set up against us. Right? Why even try? This mentality tends to cripple our desire and potential for growth and change.

It's important to realize that we are each individually responsible for our lives. Placing blame outside ourselves is really nothing more than an avoidance of responsibility and the necessary pain that comes with it. It is ultimately a detour away from the path to bliss. When we allow something to consistently hurt us, *we* are hurting ourselves. No one else is, though we often convince ourselves they are. When we accept things in our lives that are unsatisfactory, and we don't opt to make changes—don't leave that bad relationship or don't quit that horrible job—it is not fair to use those things and people as scapegoats for our reluctance to develop and progress. We must realize that we are clinging to those things, and we must examine why we haven't chosen to break those attachments, uncomfortable and unpleasant as they are. But, above all, we must realize that we *have* choices. Keeping unpleasant people or situations in our lives may be one choice we have made that has influenced us in a certain way. Other choices—like creating a nurturing set of rituals—can affect our lives in a very different way.

It is equally important to make a distinction between the forces that can really hurt us, and those we just think might. So much of the stress in our lives comes not from the actions that might cause stress, but from just the mere thought of those actions, and the subsequent fear attached to them. Fear is our greatest obstacle. Often it is much greater than anything we ever face in reality because it affects us even when there is no real danger of harm. Fear damages us on its own, whether by causing stress within our bodies, or by moving us away from necessary pain. Any step away from the discomfort of development usually leads to only greater pain. Through healthy thinking and practicing rituals that activate certain psychological responses, we can become aware of ways to bypass the mere fear of hurt and, by doing so, overcome obstacles that once stopped us or set us on a detour.

Many of the world's religions incorporate harsh physical practices designed to exorcise any fear within their followers. (Don't worry—there are none of those practices within the AVEDA rituals!) The Native Americans participate in sun dancing, a tradition in which men pierce their chests with hooks. Each man must spend five days with no food or water. Then, on the final day of this ritual, he must attach himself with the hooks and rope to a tree and break free of the hooks. The only way to do this is by throwing his weight against the ropes and tearing his skin free of the barbs. This excruciating experience is only possible once the men free themselves of fear, free themselves of this symbolic bondage to the earth and the earthly notions of pain. When they have liberated themselves in this way, those men believe they become part of the Creator.

In Indonesia, a different ritual is used to achieve oneness with God. There, people have needles inserted into their skin and go into a mental state that keeps them from bleeding when the pins are removed. Though pierced through with countless needles, they feel no pain because they are not afraid to feel pain. They don't bleed because they're not afraid they'll bleed. Though this lack of physical response is hard for us to grasp, it is a very real demonstration of the mental powers we all have the potential to achieve. Imagine possessing that degree of mind control—you can, although a lesser degree will do for our purposes here.

What these extreme examples illustrate is that so much of how we heal and grow emanates from our belief systems. We have been raised within different religious and philosophical contexts, chosen most likely by our parents and our parents' parents. No matter what religion you were raised in or have chosen for yourself, practicing your faith is a good way to promote healing. Nearly all religions speak of the importance of the will of the self, and of faith when it comes to leading a fulfilled life. You will find your most important tools in making AVEDA rituals work for you—believing in yourself, your choices, and your realized intentions—are the keys to the vehicle that drives you directly to the zone of bliss.

REFLECT

Every entrepreneur knows the importance of constantly resetting and adjusting goals, and examining his or her business's progress toward those goals on a daily basis. Similarly, each person's daily life requires the same degree of organization, planning, and analysis. That's why I call my approach to living "the business of being." Business is a process of transactions, a transfer of energy in the form of money, goods, or action. Our lives are full of such daily activities. Each one of us needs to be the leader of how they unfold. To do so, we must be conscious of our path and our mission actively to become the personal success we envision.

I have been developing what I call "the business of being" for many years, and I continually change it as I learn new practices and habits from different teachers. It began when I started meditating and keeping a diary in 1968, and then it grew out of my life experiences and my exposure to various masters. Prior to that, I had never written things down or examined my emotions. Suddenly, I was writing every day and reading my notes from the days before. It was then that I began to see a cause-and-effect relationship between my actions and my emotions. I began to analyze the cause-and-effect relationships in all the areas of my life, the way that an entrepreneur analyzes all the facets of a business.

A few years later, in the early seventies, I added another layer to the process: setting goals. It is not enough just to examine our actions and learn what *not* to do again or what to repeat. We need to rise to new levels and guide ourselves there. I have found goal setting to be a very big key to success and contentment. I have worked on my goals on a daily basis for many years, and every one of them has manifested. Still, I am never done. Out of each goal grows another. It is a continuum.

Think of your life as an organization, and become more mindful of all your thoughts, words, emotions, and actions. Imagine your life is a shop, and you are the shopkeeper. At the end of the day, the smart shopkeeper conducts an inventory. He or she doesn't just look at the computer printouts of what's been scanned as sold that day, but talks to every member of the team about their contributions. The shopkeeper then considers how effective the store's strategies and team members are, and adjusts his or her plans to keep the things that are working, and to eliminate or change the things that aren't.

This is what we need to do on a daily basis, and preferably more than once a day, in our personal lives. We need to take inventory often, so that we can remain conscious of all the relationships in our lives—the connections between our mind, body, and spirit; between our actions and our goals; between our surroundings and ourselves—and adjust them as needed. You can also use the analogy of the athlete here. This self-observation is like what professional athletes do after they play a game: With their coaches, they watch the instant replay to see what they can improve, and what is working well for them. Mirroring is like watching your day, your week, or your year, in instant replay.

Another relationship—the relationship between thoughts, words, actions, and our emotions—is one we must be highly aware of when we approach mirroring. In the business of being, the energy that is transacted is not money, but action. We each possess tremendous power over our lives and the people and happenings we meet and experience. We may not realize it, but our thoughts, hopes, and dreams become reality through the business of being, through that transaction of energy called will, or intention. A thought is a powerful thing. Give a thought words, by either putting it down on paper in a diary or saying it out loud, and that thought has even more power. By expressing your thoughts verbally or in writing, you often give them enough power to move on to the next level and materialize into an action.

Mirroring allows you to evaluate the thoughts and actions of the past and consider the ones you'll need for the future. It gives you the space to observe your actions and intentions, and to contemplate ways to manifest those intentions. It is a practice that you can do anywhere, any time to further increase the power of your ideas. I suggest you find a creative space for it, a place where you can slow down time in the morning and the evening and reflect on yourself. Maybe there's a corner of a room or a place outside where you feel you can make a private, comfortable space for yourself. You can also perform mirroring in a mirror by talking to your image and seeing yourself put your thoughts into words, into plans for action.

Relax

When you are ready to mirror, sit in your chosen place and move into a slow breathing mode, close to what is called the alpha state, where your body and your heartbeat are just above where they'd be if you were meditating or in a deep sleep. Controlled breath is our body's own natural tranquilizer. It allows us to relax our heart, all the cells of our body, and our mind.

Breath

Calming your breath can be achieved a variety of ways, the simplest of which is to breathe extra slowly, exhaling twice as long as you inhale. Make sure your breaths are deep. We have become upper-chest breathers, but the most effective breathing for meditation—and for constant awareness in our lives—is diaphragmatic. This is breathing that starts well below the chest, in the diaphragm. It changes the body chemistry, creating a very nurturing environment, which is a perfect state for effective contemplation.

Everyone can do this type of breathing. You can enhance it with the practice of the simple exercise of lying on the floor with two or three heavy books on your stomach. Breathing in such a way helps you to focus on and strengthen the diaphragm as the source of your breath. Diaphragmatic breathing will become natural. The more you practice, the easier it will be to breathe this way on a regular basis. I have been practicing diaphragmatic breathing for so many years now that it has almost become autonomic or unconscious for me. When I don't breath deeply automatically, and I activate it consciously—such as after a meeting that might not have gone the way I would have liked it to—I can feel its calming effects immediately.

Focus

When we are still, when we calm our breath, we can hear our minds and our souls best. In this state, bring to the front of your mind the goings-on in your life. To this contemplation introduce real, concrete goals, even though you know you are constantly going to change and adjust them. Every human being has got to have a strategy for life. It's a good idea even to write down times and dates. Where do you want to be tomorrow, next month, next year, when you are thirty, forty, fifty, sixty? Take a survey of the long- and short-term goals you'd like to achieve.

This is when I study my physical activities, my mental activities, all the activities between myself and other people. I reflect on my outside relationships as well as my inside relationships. I try to identify the things that represent pain, understand them, and work through that pain on the way to bliss. I try to identify the things that represent bliss and plan to continue doing those things. I encourage you to do the same.

You'll be amazed how much easier it is to stick to your goals and see results when you promote consciousness through mirroring. There's nothing to be afraid of failing to accomplish. There are no judgments. No one is keeping score. It's just you helping you.

You may want to keep a diary, so that you can efficiently keep track of your goals and your progress, your routes to pain and bliss. Your daily regimen of rituals is something to reflect on here, too. What in your routine is working for you, and what isn't? Look at all of these issues regularly and fine-tune them.

I like to take time out for mirroring three times a day. I try to do it in the morning, around noon, and again in the evening before I go to bed. Of course, there are days when I don't mirror three times a day, or even once. I should. We all should. I do my best on a daily basis, but I am not too hard on myself if a day goes by without mirroring. You also have to allow for flexibility, and not give up your rituals altogether just because you fall out of habit for a short period.

Once you have developed your own ritual of mirroring—whether it's jotting down goals after meditation, or talking to yourself in the bathroom mirror—you should add it to your daily routine, practicing it one to three times a day. Incorporating this honesty regarding your aims and achievements with yourself and others is a key to a better quality of life.

We can also add broader mirroring rituals, for monthly, seasonal, or annual inventory. I like to take stock about twice a year by removing myself from my regular environment, cleansing my body internally, and mirroring through an extended silence of about ten days. I do my best self-observation when I take a ten-day silence. I have made a tradition of doing this in India, in the mountains, about once a year. During my silence, I write a lot—about what I am pleased with in my life, what I want to change, and what my new goals are. At that time, I see how well my daily mirroring has worked. You may want to consider adding a similar practice to your annual schedule.

REDEFINE YOUR LIFE

A very important principle in mirroring and any reflection is viewing your experiences in terms of pain and bliss, rather than good and bad, or right and wrong. A key to growth is never labeling actions as right or wrong. We must not judge our thoughts, words, and actions harshly through a black-and-white lens. Our choices aren't inherently "right" or "wrong." Those judgmental views are often imposed by fear and conditioning, and they serve only to put us in a defensive mode, leading us to make future choices that aren't based on our own experiences. If we constantly look to the outside world for our clues on how to behave, we wind up in a reactive mode rather than an active mode in our own lives. Not creating our own standards, we discriminate against things that might have otherwise contributed to our bliss because we have learned from outside judgments to fear those things.

LIFE SUPPORT

A lot of what we need to grow toward fulfillment we already know. Our cells, our bodies, the larger body—the Earth—all know exactly what they need to survive and to thrive. Each one of our hearts and bodies knows very well the difference between those things that nurture them and those things that put stress on them. We must make an effort to be silent for a short time each day to listen to the very wise messages our hearts and bodies send us.

But our instincts and our own personal experiences mustn't be the only source of learning and support in our lives. We need to draw knowledge, awareness, and motivation from people outside of ourselves, people who

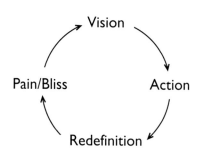

LEARN FROM PAIN—
CHOOSE BLISS

Fear, as I will say many times in this book, is the greatest obstacle to bliss. When we discriminate against thoughts, actions, or people, we are reacting with fear to what those things mean to us within ourselves. Ultimately, we are creating fear, in the form of hate, against ourselves, which leads to emotions that work against our healthy body chemistry. It is better to take situations at face value, and describe them in terms of the feelings they evoke within us personally, with words such as hot, cold, tired, lonely, happy, and energized, rather than as good or bad. All of our choices are just part of a process, and when we mirror and pay conscious attention to which elements around us evoke feelings of pain within us and which evoke bliss, we can make new choices that are uniquely suited to each one of us as individuals. These wise choices promote health and balance on all levels.

have made it their business to know more about particular aspects of wellness than we possibly can in this world of information explosion. It is important to get support from these people, whom I describe in a variety of ways—as teachers, coaches, mentors, trainers, gurus, and practitioners. Because the business of being incorporates so many different areas of focus, we need a variety of these leaders in our lives, who can give us the guidance and motivation we need on our path to bliss.

What I am talking about here is enlightenment—finding credible, learned people and letting them shed important light on the many different aspects of being. I don't mean to recommend following anyone blindly. Before choosing a mentor, or coach, get to know this person not only through his or her words and writings, but through his or her actions. Even then, bear in mind that your individual needs may vary from what your coach prescribes. Adapt to what feels good to you, but the minute something doesn't feel right, listen to yourself—to your heart and body. Your heart and body will know what is right for you. Look to others for a variety of choices, but never forget that you are your main teacher.

But bearing that in mind, I think we need many advisers. I have always sought spiritual advisers, inside and outside the faith I was raised in, which was Catholicism. I have been educated by Yogis, Buddhists, Jews, Hindus, Muslims, and many indigenous peoples. I have found that at the core, all of these belief systems hold the same kernel of truth: that it is honesty of spirit and acceptance of others that are most important. These can, and often do, exist outside of organized religion, too. Spirituality can be very personal and individual and does not necessarily require the leadership principles of religion.

In my travels I have also discovered that beyond the cities, in the forests and mountains of every continent, the local leaders practice healing through a combination of faith, plants, and foods. They are both psychologists and physiologists, which is a very holistic, integrated approach to health. So, while the languages, garments, and skin colors may be different from one culture to the next, the emphasis on truth and nature are universal to all spiritual practice.

We also need good medical advisers, such as doctors who integrate Western and indigenous medicine along with modern scientific plant medicines. We all need elements of both approaches to health in order to approach wellness holistically. There is wisdom in both traditions, and the medical field is now realizing that the two complement each other. For all my own leanings toward natural healing through plants and herbs and simple ancient traditions, I also go to Dr. Don Hensrud, a so-called Western doctor at the Mayo Clinic in Rochester, Minnesota, as well as Dr. David Simon at the Chopra Clinic in La Jolla, California, both of whom incorporate natural healing traditions and plant-derived medicines. For some things we need surgery, or pharmaceuticals, in order to help our bodies make effective use of naturopathic remedies.

Physical coaches are important, too. Yoga instructors help us work through difficult postures and get the most out of stretching, physically and spiritually. As for more strenuous activity, even if we're aware of a good mode of exercise, we often need the coach to say, "Okay, let's go! Let's go out and kick some balls, and stretch some muscles." If you can't afford to work with trainers like these on your own, you can join a class. Participating in classes is also a very good way to be motivated by other people.

You can also learn from people around you who just seem to be doing things right. If you don't have people in your life who you feel set good examples, reach beyond your inner circle and meet new people from whom you can cull wisdom, guidance, and support. Everybody out there is a potential teacher. But most of all, we are our own ultimate teachers. We must learn to recognize and trust the lessons our bodies, minds, hearts, and souls are encouraging us to learn.

STILL WATERS RUN DEEP

Meditation is a ritual that I recommend as part of everyone's daily routine. The word *meditation* is a very broad term. People have strong associations with and assumptions regarding this word, and often those ideas intimidate them from trying this practice out for themselves. They have heard it means clearing your mind completely and they rightfully determine that is nearly impossible to do. We simply cannot think of nothing. So, they figure it's not for them. Or they believe meditation is only valid if it's done for a certain length of time, which just isn't true. If you have tried meditation before, or this is your first encounter with it, try to free your mind of all the things you've heard about it. Let's look at it anew.

What is meditation? When people ask me what kind of meditation I practice, I always have to smile. It's as if people assume meditation is a type of religion, and they're asking what type of religion I practice. Meditation is not a religion. But every religion that I'm familiar with incorporates meditation in some form. So, back to the question: What is meditation? Meditation to me is transcending your daily flow of thoughts to focus on one thought as long as possible. It involves contemplating that thought, knowing the meaning of that thought, and then putting energy behind that thought. Meditation is concentration with surrender, and with controlled, relaxed breathing. If I coordinate, or synergize my breath with a thought, this observation helps me stay centered on that idea for much longer than I ever could with no breath control.

Visualization is another component of meditation. We can visualize the things we want, or we can visualize things that arouse positive thoughts and a nurturing feeling within ourselves. Visualizing the things we want is one step toward making those things real in our lives, making them manifest.

We can use it to help our bodies fight off disease. One oncologist whom I admire, Dr. Carl Simonton, teaches his cancer patients visualization techniques to use along with the radiation therapy he gives them. He instructs them to visualize their bodies conquering the cancer as their white blood cells attack cancer cells, or to envision themselves perfectly well. Many of his patients have helped their bodies to produce white blood cells necessary to eliminate tumors within their bodies. The visualization techniques are also used by his patients to help combat the nausea and other side effects often associated with chemotherapy.

But we can tap into the benefits of visualization when we are well, too. This practice can help us achieve goals. I always find that those things that I want and visualize come to me after I let go of my attachment to them. If I visualize what I want and then let go and get on with other things, in time, what I envisioned comes to me. Or we can use it to nurture peace in ourselves. To create a positive state of mind, I visualize something I love, a rose, for example. Because I love roses, they represent to me an image that is

The divine rose provides soothing, cooling, and relaxing gifts for the body, mind, and spirit.

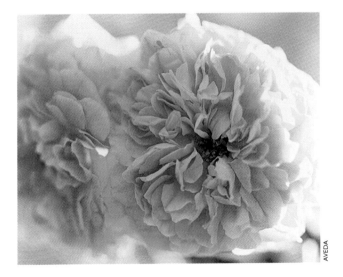

AVEDA

divine. When I contemplate a rose, inhaling and exhaling slowly, it gives me a truly divine feeling, which allows me to operate from a balanced, centered place of contentment. The image of a rose reminds me of joy, and that frees me from any anger and pain I may be holding on to at that moment. Focusing on things that make you laugh is another option in meditation. Humor and laughter create joy and evoke physical and chemical changes in the body that promote well-being. You can use any and all of these variations of meditation and visualization to increase your health and happiness on a daily basis.

Some people like to go to a special spot, which they've set up just for meditation, maybe with pillows and a certain amount of light, or a candle, to focus on and help them concentrate. Other people can do it anywhere—on their lunch break, in a quiet office, or even in a restaurant full of people. In the AVEDA Institute in Minneapolis, I have set up a room just for contemplation and meditation, where instructors and students can take restorative breaks. I think every office would benefit from such a spot. Periods of silent contemplation throughout the day would do wonders for people's attention spans and productivity levels in the workplace.

I recommend including meditation, once or twice daily, in your set of rituals. No matter what the details of your particular meditation ritual may be, this practice can help you balance your state of being and achieve your goals. After meditation, one is "grounded" emotionally and physically, and so it's a great time for mirroring and goal setting. When you're done, make sure to give thanks—to your self, to the larger collective self that includes you, and to whatever divinities you believe in.

A BREATH OF FRESH AIR

Certainly we all know how to breathe. We don't even need to give any thought to autonomic breathing—our bodies take care of that. Inhalation and exhalation are our most basic human functions, and the most vital to our very life. If there is no breath, there is death.

But there are more dimensions to breath than are readily obvious. Breath is an important link in the mind-body relationship. Scientists have documented that when our breath is calm, our mind is calm. There is also another parallel that doctors in a recent Pennsylvania study have discovered when looking at our brain-wave patterns: We can sustain our concentration on one thought only for the length of one inhalation and exhalation. With each new breath we take, a new thought enters the mind.

Therefore, when we meditate, it is important to slow down our breath. We do this in order to avoid jerking our minds from one thought to another very quickly. If we want to keep our minds from wandering as we meditate, it is key to keep our breath from racing.

Not only good for meditation, controlled, slow breathing is also a wonderful weapon we can use any time to battle stress. When a person is calm and breathing is slow, effective, and steady, the body is in a nurtured state, which strengthens the immune system. Quite simply, healthy breathing is key to the body's ability to heal itself.

What is meant by "effective" breath? It is a slow, deep, complete breath. When we inhale deeply, allowing a new gust of oxygen to fill our body cavity from the bottom on up, and then exhale slowly, from the diaphragm, we are practicing a very cleansing, nurturing form of breathing that helps our bodies eliminate stress and toxins. Take a moment to try this type of breathing now. Do you feel how your body relaxes, each muscle falling into its natural, comfortable position? You were probably a bit tense before you took this breath, but most likely didn't even know it. Bringing this consciousness to our breath gives it the power to relieve strain and heal us.

We need to heal ourselves from the impact of stress nearly every day. No matter how healthy a life we lead, there will always be stress acting on our minds and bodies—from the environment, from our jobs, from our relationships, and even from our food. This is the main reason we need a set of daily holistic rituals. We need to manage and eliminate stress regularly because it is harmful to our beings, and because it can accumulate. If we do not let go of stress, then we keep piling it up and our bodies' circuitry becomes overloaded, making us perpetually tense.

There are different types of controlled breathing we can use for different effects. I have just introduced you to a calming one. Others are meant to invigorate the body. In the second part of the book, I'll talk more specifically about breathing exercises for enhancing each.

SAY A LITTLE PRAYER

We are all raised with different faiths, organized and personal. Whether you're a devout Christian, Jew, Muslim, Buddhist, Hindu, or you just sense there's a power greater than us out there, I believe that practicing your faith and strengthening the spiritual portion of your life will help you achieve bliss. More important than the specifics of what you believe is that you believe in something. However you worship, whatever you worship, don't abandon it just because you've taken up meditation. Each religion has its own form of meditation, which might be different from the mirroring and meditation you have added to your daily routine. I recommend doing both, because believing in all the spiritual forces that support us fuels our commitment to a healthy lifestyle and enhances the many positive results of our nurturing habits.

THE SWEET SMELL OF SUCCESS

Whether it comes in the remembered scent of a flower-filled garden where you played as a child, bread baking in your mother's kitchen, or the mist from the ocean where you spent a blissful summer vacation, we all know the transporting and transcending powers of these familiar, happy smells. One whiff, and our minds take us away from our current cares and concerns, back to the warm and fuzzy moments when we first experienced them. Briefly, we relive that happy moment, experiencing all love and no fear. This powerful, transporting experience is the basis for the magic of aromatherapy. By exposing ourselves to plant and flower essences that arouse nurturing feelings in us, we can manipulate our brain chemistry to affect our behavior in a positive way. When we surround ourselves with the scents that inspire creativity within us, we are more creative. When we surround ourselves with the scents that inspire confidence in us, we are more confident. And so on. Which scents evoke these emotions? They're different for everyone, based on our sense memories. While plants do have some inherent properties that give them invigorating or relaxing and hot or cold properties, that plays only a small role in arousing certain feelings within us. It's the loving, nurturing thoughts *brought on by the scents,* based on our prior associations with them, that activate our emotions and our brain chemistry.

All of our sensory experiences, from birth on, are logged in our brains. Every taste, smell, sight, sound, and touch each of us has ever encountered is in our mind's database, along with our reaction to it, be it comfort or pain. That first time we burned our finger on the stove our minds registered pain. As a result, now, when we touch hot things, our brains provide the sensation of pain seconds before our flesh and nerves have come to that conclusion. In some cases, just the thought of touching something burning hot provides us with a strong sense memory.

"Sense memory" is a powerful tool we can all tap into. Method actors use it very effectively to evoke familiar emotions on the stage or screen. They re-create experiences in their minds so that they can develop the

AROMATHERAPY IMPOSTERS

If you were to visit the corporate headquarters of Aveda in Minneapolis, you wouldn't hear the word "aromatherapy" uttered too often. That might seem surprising since aromatics are such an important aspect of Aveda products. But aromatherapy is a word that frequently has been misappropriated and overused, and, as a result, has lost its true meaning. These days, anything that has been dressed up with synthetic perfumes is marketed as being useful for aromatherapy, from bubble bath to scented waste basket liners. It's kind of like the word "natural," which has been diluted by the corporate marketing machine to include just about anything that isn't made of plastic.

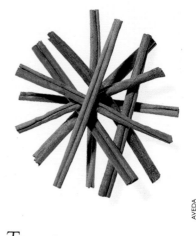

AVEDA

The smell of soothing scents like cinnamon deeply nurtures us.

WHAT "AROMATHERAPY" REALLY MEANS

Instead of aromatherapy, at AVEDA we say "pure plant aromaology-therapy," because we know that fragrances aren't truly therapeutic to our body chemistry if they're not derived from plants. Synthetic fragrances can fool our noses momentarily, but not our brains or the rest of the cells in our bodies, which are much too discerning and intelligent to fall for impostor scents. In the grander scheme of things, how therapeutic can synthetic fragrances be if they're harmful to our environment when they're manufactured, and later, when they're used?

Yet although "Pure-fume" and "pure plant aromaology-therapy" are distinctions I coined, I realize the latter is quite a mouthful. In this book, I'll stick with aromatherapy, the term with which we're all much more familiar. But know that when I use it, I'm referring *strictly* to those essences and oils that are pure plant derivatives. And think about it the next time you see the word *aromatherapy* on a candle or a jar of bath salts. Read the ingredients. Your whole olfactory system will thank you for choosing the ones that are pure.

appropriate, authentic reactions for an audience. Through aromatherapy, each of us can engage in method living, using natural plant- and flower-based scents to bring about familiar, desired emotional states at will. Our minds already have vast stores of information regarding which scents motivate us, which scents make us feel loved, which scents make us feel creative, or empowered, or hungry, or agitated, or satisfied.

We can add to that library of stimuli by introducing new scents during nurturing practices so we'll have additional positive references to draw upon. For example, diffuse some tangerine, marjoram, lavender, citronella, pennyroyal, or eucalyptus oil in the room while you meditate and visualize your goals. Over time, just the scent of natural tangerine will put you into a motivated state. To take full advantage of the powerful, improving influence of aromatherapy, I recommend taking what I call a sensory journey to discover which scents, by their own nature, produce feelings of love within you. You can take this journey at an AVEDA store, where there are thirty-two essences to experience, or at a health food store or a nursery, with an herbalist or on your own.

You may wonder why I keep saying that the scents we use should be natural, plant- and flower-derived ones. The market is full of synthetic perfume–scented incense, candles, deodorants, air fresheners, household cleansers, soaps, lotions, and oils, which are much cheaper than natural ones, and convincing enough to fool our noses. The plant's interior chemist is superior to the human chemist every time. Each plant has millions of years of intelligence and experience that can be imitated but not duplicated by humans. All we do when we imitate nature is pollute it; so we need to cultivate and sustain nature rather than imitate it. Each of us can take part in the cultivation process by growing plants and flowers in our living and working environments.

When we smell a synthetic facsimile of a plant essence, initially, our emotional memory will give us a short-term pleasing effect. But that's it. An artificial scent won't be as effective in the long run as its natural counterpart. What's more, the petrochemicals used more often than not in these synthetic scents put stress on our bodies. While synthetic aromas may smell great, when we use them we are breathing in toxins that our bodies must then work to remove. True aromatherapy removes stresses; it does not create new ones within our bodies, not to mention the environment. Petrochemicals pollute when they're produced and when we use them outside the Earth's crust. Besides, the body of the Earth needs the oil from which petrochemicals are derived. Removing that part of the Earth's body as we have been doing is like removing our spleen or pancreas, or some other vital part of our body.

Plants and natural plant essences also have more to offer than just their lovely aromas and natural chemical properties. They carry antiseptic qualities as well. They keep the body and the environment around it pure. Plant-derived essences, and the emotions they arouse, can aid the healing process in other ways, too. In the second half of this book, I'll talk more specifically about ways we can use aromatherapy, and particular essences, to enhance daily nurturing habits.

PURE AND NATURAL

The importance of purity is not limited to those substances that we breathe. For the same reasons that we should use natural plant and flower essences in our aromatherapy, we should also incorporate them into our cleansers, moisturizers, sunscreens, and hair-care and makeup products. Many plant essences have incredible molecular potency, which is very useful for personal hygiene and household cleaning. They are antiseptic, as well as antifungal, antiyeast, antiparasite, antiviral, and antibacterial. They are fine insect repellents as well. By including essential oils in our cleansing and beauty products, we can combine the benefits of healthy hygiene and cosmetics with aromatherapy, giving ourselves a little extra nurturing as we clean the house, bathe, receive a massage, or even style our hair. It is most healthy to expose our bodies to the intelligence of nature with everything that touches them, including body washes, soaps, shampoos, lipsticks, shaving creams, massage oils, and even substances like laundry detergents and household cleansers. For the benefit of our bodies and the world, I recommend using products with low or no concentrations of petrochemicals, and high concentrations of natural plant essences, wherever possible.

THE MAGIC TOUCH

For those who have not included massage as part of your regular daily life thus far, the idea of getting one on a daily basis must sound like a tremendous luxury. For many of us, the word *massage* brings to mind a pampering environment, like a spa or salon, and a professional masseur. That's a good image, and it's something we should all indulge in as often as we can afford to. However, many do not have the means to afford this sort of professional treatment every day, week, or month. But that doesn't mean we can't be massaged every single day of our lives. I recommend practicing self-massage and trading massages with a partner, if you have one, as part of your

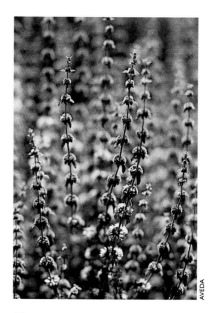

*P*ennyroyal provides a motivating fragrance.

THE SCIENCE OF FEELINGS

The Western medical community perceived the idea that emotions greatly affect our physical health as little more than a theory for many years. That was until a brilliant scientist, Dr. Candace Pert, found a way to scientifically explain and document this phenomenon. Through her research into immunity, Dr. Pert has manifested evidence of the communication between the psyche and all the cells of the body. She explains this biochemical correspondence in her groundbreaking book *The Molecules of Emotion*, a fascinating read which I highly recommend. In essence, she has documented what the yogis in the Himalayas, the shamans, and the medicine men from around the world have known for ages: that a sound mind really is the key to a sound body.

HOW THE BODY FEELS

At the root of Dr. Pert's findings is a molecule, situated on the surface of cells in the brain and certain parts of the body, called the opiate receptor. Dr. Pert discovered this molecule in the early seventies. She explains in her book that receptors are very rare, complicated molecules, made up of proteins and amino acids, which function as sensors. They wait for messages from other cells—but they must be the right messages. Receptors are like keyholes that way. Once the right molecules, known as *ligands,* come along, bearing the right messages, the receptor and the ligand join forces. The ligand is able to enter the molecule's host cell and to alter it positively. The cell becomes stronger and immune to illnesses. Dr. Pert gives this very simple explanation of this relationship:

"If the cell is the engine that drives all life, then the receptors are the buttons on the control panel of that engine, and a specific ligand is the finger that pushes that button and gets things started."

daily routine. These massages cost nothing and are highly beneficial on many levels.

There is nothing frivolous about getting massaged. It is actually a very accessible and serious therapy, in terms of its ability to remove toxins, increase circulation, and strengthen immunity. In fact, Dr. Candace B. Pert, Ph.D., research professor in the Department of Physiology and Biophysics at Georgetown University, has done research that shows regular massaging leads to stronger immune systems. Her work demonstrates that people who are massaged every day go into a regular deep state of nurturing and relaxation during this time, sparking the production of neuropeptides, or immune system building blocks. These natural substances contribute to the body's defense system that is in turn better able to fend off any illness or stress it might encounter from day to day.

We can give ourselves these benefits by practicing breathing and massage from head to toe, on ourselves, or with our partners.

In the second half of the book, I'll suggest guidelines for a simple self-massage you can do each morning and/or evening, as well as tips for massages by and for a partner. This doesn't have to take up a tremendous amount of time. You can give yourself a massage in a matter of five or ten minutes; you and a partner can give each other twenty-minute to hour-long massages, depending upon how much time you have available.

In addition to these massage practices, there's a mind-breath exercise that I like to include in my daily rituals called the 61-point exercise. With this exercise you can actually stimulate all the pressure points on your body through visualization and breathing. By doing so, you activate the flow of energy in your body and break up all the blockages that stress can erect.

The 61-point exercise takes about twenty minutes and its therapeutic value is well worth the time. Performing it is quite simple. With each inhalation and exhalation focus your attention on a different point on your body, working through all sixty-one. This is an easy, beneficial exercise that involves reliving nurturing moments. I urge you to try it.

BODIES IN MOTION

The 61-point exercise will help you condition both your mind and body to some extent. But other forms of motion and exercise are very important if you are striving to reach optimal body function as well as "yoga"—or the union of mind, body, and spirit.

Just as there are those breathing techniques that calm the body and

THE ENERGY BATH

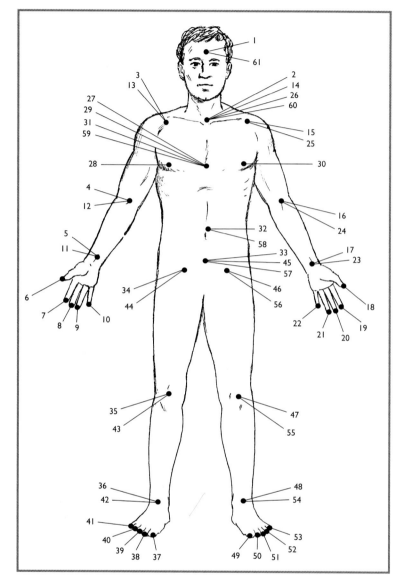

A.K.A. THE 61-POINT EXCERCISE

1. Lie down and relax in a comfortable spot.
2. Close your eyes and breathe from your diaphragm in smooth, even breaths.
3. Concentrate on each of the points, starting from 1 in the center of the forehead, for about 30 seconds.
4. As you come to a new spot envision a star or bright light emanating from it. See that light glow brightly until you move to the next.
5. When you have hit all 61 points, concentrate on lighting all of them at once. Bathe in this healing energy.
6. As you finish, take a few moments to enjoy the deep relaxation you feel.

THE 61-POINT RELAXATION'S FOUR DEFINITE BENEFITS

Physical Relaxation

By lying flat on the floor and concentrating on the breath, all of the muscles of the body are allowed to relax. This conscious physical relaxation is important for revitalization as it allows to body to rest in a way not comparable to sleep.

Mental Focus

The ability to focus eludes many people. We often hear about the short attention span prevalent in today's society. The 61-point relaxation teaches the mind to focus. By keeping the attention of the mind on each of the points and only the points, the mind is learning to focus. Focus helps one achieve all of his or her goals and dreams—physical, mental, and spiritual.

Integration of the Left and Right Hemispheres of the Brain

The 61-point relaxation engages the activities of both the left and right sides of the brain. The left brain, or analytical side, is used by the counting in numerical order of the points 1 through 61. The right brain, or creative side, is used to visualize a bright-colored star at each of the points. By utilizing both hemispheres of the brain, the body is learning balance.

Inwardness

The inward attention achieved through the 61-point relaxation increases self-awareness and teaches us to pay attention to the internal workings of the body. This knowledge is priceless in regard to self-healing. This subtle exercise can bring about the same effects as acupuncture purely through the energy directed to points on the body by thought alone.

HAPPY = HEALTHY

Among the ligands that can latch on to opiate receptors are peptides, tiny pieces of proteins that have been recognized as the first materials of life. The best fingers to push those receptor buttons on cells in the brain and body turn out to be something called neuropeptides. Dr. Pert says they are the building blocks of immunity.

The cells of the brain are rich in neuropeptides. In fact, it is in the parts of the brain that control emotion in which the highest concentration of neuropeptides sit. They are produced in higher quantities when there is a low level of stress and a high perception of nurturance. Very simply, when we feel happy, our brains and certain body parts produce more neuropeptides, making them available to the opiate receptors of more cells, leaving more cells fortified with immunity. The sternum, in the chest, is another area where neuropeptides are produced. And so massaging this area regularly can increase immunity, too.

others that invigorate it, there are various forms of body movement that have different effects on our metabolism as well. Most of us need each day to engage in both calming and invigorating motion to reach our highest mind and body function.

There are many calming forms of movement that are derived from ancient traditions, such as yoga, tai chi, and some of the Asian martial arts. A more modern calming mode of exercise is called Pilates and relies upon the strength of our minds to help us push past our previously assumed strength boundaries.

Invigorating modes of movement include more aerobic activities, like running and walking, participating in aerobics classes, weight lifting, playing tennis, and working out on cardiovascular machines such as a cross-country skier, a stair climber, a stationary bicycle, a treadmill, and others.

It is important to remember in this competitive age that even when you're engaged in aerobic activities, you should set a comfortable pace for yourself, one at which you can still practice healthy breathing, through your nose. The nose is an important filter of the air we inhale. I once heard a yogi say that if you find you need to breathe through your mouth while you're exercising, then you're overextending yourself. It is a good rule to live and moderate yourself by.

In the second half of the book, I'll go into more detail on different options for calming and invigorating exercise, and I'll recommend some for different times of the day. I'll also touch on body types, based on the ancient elements of earth, wind, fire, and water, and which exercises will work best with regard to those.

YOU ARE WHAT YOU EAT

The ancient intelligence regarding body types of Ayurveda has a lot to contribute when we talk about diet.

While we all manifest characteristics of all three body types, known in Ayurveda as *vatta*, *pitta*, and *kapha*, we each tend to lean more toward one. For each body type, relating to the elements of earth, wind, fire, and water, there are certain recommended dietary considerations. In the second half of the book, there's a questionnaire to help you figure out to which of these you personally are more inclined. Once you've completed this questionnaire, you can help yourself to become more balanced by following some of dietary suggestions I suggest for your body type based on this Ayurvedic wisdom.

Regardless of your body type, and whatever your eating habits, I recommend strongly that you consider eating only organic foods, for the good of the smaller body, your own, as well as the larger body, the Earth. To begin with, when fruits and vegetables are treated with pesticides, they become much less nutritious. In addition, pesticides deplete the soil and the plants of important nutrients that naturally circulate when crops are allowed to grow without man-made products added. When we eat organic foods, which are harvested without pesticides, we are treated to a much greater menu of nutrients, and as a result, we absorb those and are healthier. Organic foods are a bit more expensive than foods that aren't. But it's worth the extra money to have the extra nutrients and to support the organic-farming movement. When we support organic farming, we help farmers to keep the air and the soil clean, and to provide nutrient-rich food to ourselves and others.

Now you have the mind, body, spirit overview in which you can place your daily healthy living practices. You can see how all things are interconnected and why I've incorporated elements here you may not find in other health and beauty books. Now let's look at these things a bit more closely. Let's start with Ayurveda.

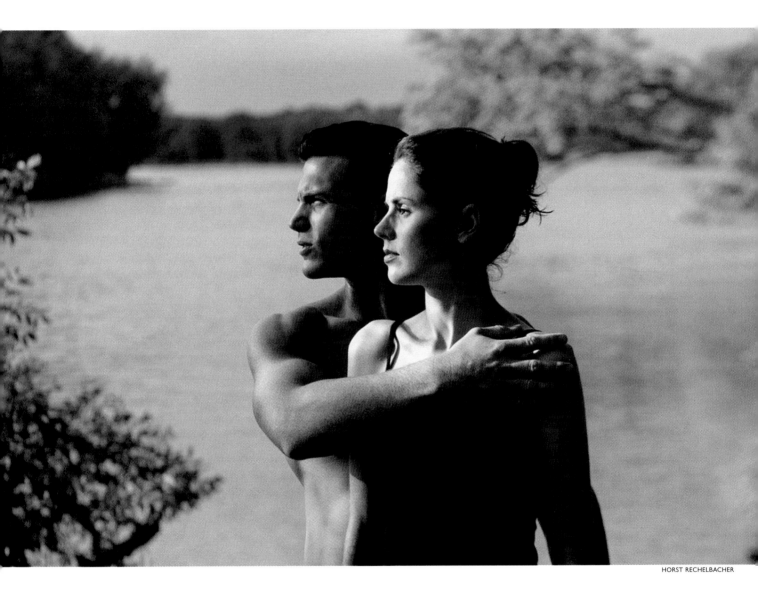

HORST RECHELBACHER

3

Ayurveda's Individual Incentives

Everyone should be his own physician. We ought to assist, and not to force, nature. Eat with moderation what agrees with your constitution. Nothing is good for the body but what we can digest. What medicine can procure digestion? Exercise. What will recruit strength? Sleep. What will alleviate incurable evils? Patience.

—Voltaire

WE ARE ALL UNIQUE. WE EACH HAVE VERY DIFFERENT constitutions, externally, internally, emotionally, and spiritually. This is due to the fact that we carry our own one-of-a-kind combinations of the elements of air, fire, earth, water, and space within each of those sectors of the self.

So, while we all share much in common, we are not the same. The idea that what's good for one person's body is also good for another's is a very limited, limiting concept of Western medicine that is gradually being abandoned by medical practitioners who have recognized the uniqueness of every human body. Our diets, health care, exercise routines, and other healthful practices are most effective when they take into account our very particular needs.

We are born with our individual constitutions, and they stay with us our entire lives. How we treat our bodies, minds, and spirits affects the balance of the elements within our highly customized makeups. There are specific foods, habits, and exercises that might promote well-being within one person, yet increase stress within another.

We can, and should, tailor our daily routines of nurturing habits to the specific needs and inclinations of each of our bodies. Before creating a routine, we each should study ourselves and our makeups so that we can most wisely choose the foods, scents, forms of movement, and other factors that will help us find our own perfect balance. The discoveries you make about yourself in this chapter will help you to incorporate informed choices from the menus of practices put forth in later chapters.

How do we figure all this out? There's a very scientific, proven method of learning what our individual constitutions are, based on the ancient wisdom of Ayurveda and other indigenous holistic traditions from around the globe. Later in this chapter you'll find a questionnaire that will help you diagnose your particular Ayurvedic makeup of the elements, and determine what foods, essential oils, and exercises work best with your nature.

Ayurveda, an approach to prevention of illness, healing, and overall well-being, is one of the oldest healing traditions in the world. It dates back more than 3,500 years to the Vedas, divine Hindu texts of knowledge from India. But it is not based merely on religion and culture. The scientific explanations and approaches to healing presented in those ancient texts are taken very seriously by the modern medical community, in both the East and the West, and, lately, often are integrated into typically Western medical practices. There are specific Ayurvedic approaches to every aspect of medicine, including surgery and psychology. Both Freud and Jung studied Ayurvedic psychology as they were formulating their own theories on the subject.

Ayurveda considers our mind, our body, and our spirit, and helps us assess what we require on all levels in order to be in balance, making it a fully integrated medical system. At the root of Ayurvedic philosophy are the five elements: air, fire, earth, water, and space. Other ancient indigenous traditions and modern practitioners of complementary medicine employ these elements as well, as they look to understand an individual's relationship to the universe, which is also made up of those five elements. Native American, African, Chinese, and Tibetan medicine are among the other practices that incorporate the five elements as the basic building blocks of everything in the universe, and the variables that determine the different characteristics each individual entity in it displays.

We all possess some of each of the five elements, but within our own compositions some are amplified, and others are subdued. This allows for the vast variety of forms that energy takes on our physical plane of existence. It will be helpful to use the Ayurvedic model of *doshas*, or certain common element combinations, to understand your own elemental makeup. The questionnaire that follows in this chapter will enable you to do just that.

THE AYURVEDIC DOSHAS AND THEIR CHARACTERISTICS

VATA	**PITTA**	**KAPHA**
composed of infinity (space) and air	*composed of fire*	*composed of earth and water*

primary functions in the body

VATA:
movement and expansion
blood and lymph circulation
neuromuscular movement
movement of food through digestive tract
respiration
nervous system

PITTA:
transformations in the body
digestion
heat
mental decisions
coloration of the skin
visual perception

KAPHA:
lubrication, structure, and support
lubrication of respiratory tract
lubrication of digestive tract
lubrication of joints
skeletal system

adjectives

VATA:
light
dry
cold

PITTA:
light
moist
hot

KAPHA:
heavy
moist
cold

additional adjectives

VATA:
changeable
quick
irregular

PITTA:
intense
sharp

KAPHA:
slow
dense
smooth
stable

physical characteristics

VATA:
light, thin build
difficulty gaining weight
thin, dry hair
tendency toward dry skin

PITTA:
medium build
tendency toward early graying or balding
tendency toward sensitive skin
strong digestion
intense eyes
good sleeper; needs less sleep than most

KAPHA:
heavy, large, or powerful build
difficulty losing weight
thick hair
smooth skin
good sleeper; needs more sleep than most

general characteristics

VATA:
strong short-term memory
moves quickly
likes to experience new things
likes to meet new people
is very creative and quick thinking
is talkative
communicates well
adapts to change
sleeps lightly

PITTA:
very intelligent
organized and precise
good decision maker
usually very focused
preference for routines
excellent teachers and speakers

KAPHA:
loving and compassionate
good long-term memory
laid back
saver of lots of different things (old clothes, money, etc.)
loyal
supportive

out-of-balance characteristics

VATA:
nervousness and anxiety
agitated mentally
worried a lot
unreliable
too talkative or too quick speech
weakened digestion

PITTA:
angry
irritable
judgmental
intimidating
cruel or harsh to others
stubborn

KAPHA:
needy
greedy
attachment to people or schedules
tendency to stay in bad relationships

IT'S ELEMENTARY

Looking to the Ayurvedic doshas, or the common element makeups, we can discover a lot about our bodies, minds, and spirits. Which category we fall into can help us determine what foods and scents we like, the climates and seasons we prefer, as well as the shapes our bodies will naturally tend toward and what our temperaments will generally be.

There are three of those common element makeups in Ayurveda, and they are often referred to as the tridoshas. The Ayurvedic names for them are as follows: vata, dominated by the elements air and space; pitta, dominated by fire; and kapha, dominated by water and earth.

We each possess aspects of all the elements and, therefore, certain amounts of the three doshas within ourselves. But we are usually more inclined toward one or two of them from birth. So, we might be considered vata, pitta, kapha, or vata-pitta, pitta-kapha, or vata-kapha, depending upon which of the elements dominates us.

One of the goals of Ayurvedic medicine is to keep our particular elemental makeups, or doshas, in balance. By doing so, we create and maintain harmony within the self, and between the self and its environment. When we treat our bodies, minds, and spirits appropriately, they are in balance. When our elemental makeups are out of balance, we become susceptible to stress and, subsequently, disease. Often, we need to choose things that are opposite to our inclinations in order to get into balance. To select only the foods, surroundings, and people that are similar to those in our doshas leads to an excess of those elements in our systems, and a subsequent imbalance. For example, a person who is dominated by the element of fire needs to eat foods that are less fiery, less hot and spicy, in order to maintain digestive well-being. A kapha person should have some pitta friends to balance his calm and steadiness with fire and energy.

We each need to have all of the five elements present in our lives, at the particular levels our systems require, in order to be in balance. The elements are present in everything—in foods, in body movements, in self-expressions, even our own body parts. Different functions of the body as well as diseases—which are interferences with certain body parts—are associated with certain elements and, therefore, with each of the doshas. For example, vata, dominated by air and space, is responsible for body flexibility. When one's vata is out of balance, he or she might experience joint pain, or arthritis.

On the previous page are some of the characteristics and functions associated with each of the three common doshas. Pay attention to them all, and bear in mind that even if one of the doshas is not dominant within your particular makeup, it still affects you to some extent since we all have at least of bit of each within us.

Vata—Air and Space

Some of the adjectives associated with vata—which rules things that are primarily dominated by the element of air—have the qualities of air. They are light, cold, dry, brittle, astringent, active, mobile, scattered, clear, irregular, and random. Vata is a dosha associated with all that is ephemeral and quick-changing. In our environment vata increases during the early winter and rainy season. Vata also dominates the afternoon and early night and, in the course of a lifetime, is strongest during old age. So during those times, we try to avoid foods and exercises with vata traits.

Likewise, people who are dominated by the vata elements of air and space have qualities our minds naturally associate with those elements. Vata people tend to be lightweight—thin. They don't eat a whole lot. Their taste prefers mostly sweet, sour, and salty foods. Their skin tends to be dry, rough, and carry a darker tone. They prefer climates that are warm and damp. Vatas are very active and don't sleep much. Some might say they're restless, and their minds are that way, too. They talk a lot, and quickly. Their short-

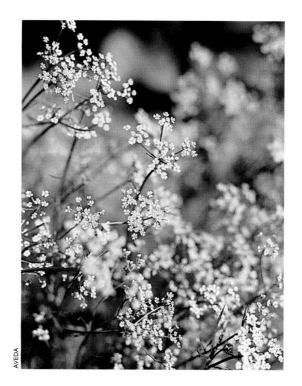

AVEDA

Caraway, a spice that balances vata—air and space elements—is stimulating and energizing.

term memories are stronger than their long-term memories, and they have a tendency to be insecure emotionally.

The vata elements are responsible for body motion, respiration, sensory impulses, autonomic mind function, circulation, separating digested from undigested food, regulation of menses, and the passage of body fluids. Consequently, it is usually a sign of vata imbalance when one experiences difficulty with those functions as indicated by such ailments as joint pain, arthritis, constipation, heart disease, menstrual disorders, blood pressure problems, and emotional imbalance. The antidotes for these illnesses stemming from vata imbalances are food, people, and activities that have the opposite properties.

The recommended diet for people dominated by the vata elements is comprised mostly of foods that are heavy and solid. It includes milk, buttermilk, okra, green beans, eggs, fish, basmati rice, oats, almonds, and sunflower seeds. Vatas should avoid the following foods, especially during the early winter and rainy season: yogurt, cabbage, cauliflower, leeks, peas, potatoes, spinach, peppers, chickpeas, kidney beans, turkey, cold drinks, and coffee.

Vata people will be inclined to engage in excessive aerobic exercise. Most long-distance runners are vatas. But vatas need also to incorporate more relaxing types of exercise, or they might take their air element out of balance, to excess.

Pitta—Fire

The word *pitta*, when translated from Sanskrit, means to heat or burn. Fittingly, the characteristics of pitta relate to the qualities of fire. Those inherent characteristics are hot, spicy, sharp, liquid, fluid, sour, slightly oily, pungent, aggressive, yellow, and blue. Pitta increases during the summer for all of us. This dosha is at its highest at midday and midnight, and, over the course of a lifetime, it is strongest during adult age, the midtwenties to the late fifties. During those times, we all should try to avoid foods and exercise regimens with pitta traits so as not to create an excess of fire and water within ourselves.

People dominated by the pitta element, fire, manifest physical and behavioral characteristics that resemble them. For example, pittas tend to get hot and sweaty easily. They have color in their skin; sometimes this manifests itself in the form of pink cheeks or freckles. They like cool climates, and have strong appetites for spicy, sweet, and bitter foods. Their eyes get red easily. Pittas can be fierce in their anger, and it's easy to get their ire up.

CONFESSIONS OF A PITTA-KAPHA

For better and for worse, I am a pitta-kapha, or fire-earth type. There are many wonderful elements to this makeup, but as with any dosha combination, when it gets out of balance, things get difficult.

My mother was a pitta-kapha, too, and my father was a pitta-vata, very thin and fast-moving. So there was no way for me to escape the pitta influence.

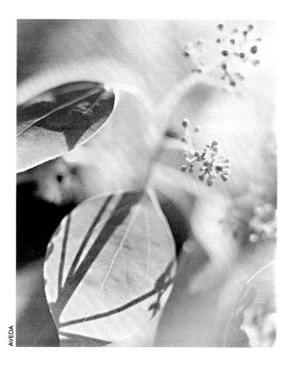

AVEDA

Camphor calms the pitta—fire element. It can soothe throat and lung ailments no matter what your dominant dosha.

BALANCING PITTA

Pitta is my strongest dosha. It is what gives me my drive as a creator and entrepreneur. My positive experience with my pitta element is that it gives me tremendous enthusiasm to create things and to get people together to activate a plan. It is the fire in my belly. But on the flip side, when things don't go according to my plan, that fire element causes me to erupt like a volcano. The up side to that is the fact that I let it all out and then move on. The downside is that I sometimes injure people around me with my words and my temper. Then apologies are in order. I often look at this side of myself in my daily inventory and try to make changes.

Over the years, through my self-observation and self-coaching, I have definitely improved in balancing my pitta. But there's always work to be done. I try to eat foods that keep the fire element in balance—not too much spicy, hot food. I do breathing exercises geared toward calming my mind and body. I like to avoid staying out in hot weather; I sweat at all times of the year, as it is. And I go for long, fast walks, but I don't exercise too vigorously because that gets me overheated and puts the fire element out of balance again.

They tend to be emotionally intense. Articulate and precise people with strong memories, pittas make great entrepreneurs and other sorts of leaders.

The pitta element is responsible for our vision, digestion, heat production, metabolism, immunity, the color of our skin, our organs and our body fluids, appetite, thirst, body suppleness, and intellectual thought. When pitta is out of balance, there are problems with those functions, such as vision impairments, yellowness of eyes, high- or low-grade body temperatures, yellow discoloration of body fluids, jaundice of skin, and confusion. The antidotes for illnesses stemming from pitta imbalances are people, places, and things that have the opposite properties.

People with a predominantly pitta constitution should stick to foods that are less spicy in order to help achieve and maintain balance. They should include in their diet such foods as milk, butter, apples, avocado, watermelon, sweet plums, lettuce, okra, cabbage, spinach, eggs, fish, chicken, chickpeas, wheat, rice, and oats. Among the foods they should avoid, especially during the summer when pitta is high, are yogurt, sour cream, lemons, bananas, papaya, garlic, leeks, radishes, almonds, cashew nuts, peppers, chilies, and other hot and spicy foods.

Moderate aerobic activity, such as walking at a medium to fast pace, is recommended for people with pitta constitutions, although people of all doshas should design a personal exercise regimen that includes a balance of both calming and invigorating movement.

Kapha—Earth and Water

Kapha is the elemental makeup that has the greatest solidity to it, physically and emotionally. It is the dosha of permanence, or slow change. Words used to describe kapha characteristics are heavy, cool, soft, thick, viscous, firm, stable, sweet, and slimy. Kapha is heightened in the winter of every year and in our youth. During those times, we should try to avoid foods and exercise routines that have kapha traits, so as not to create an excess of water and earth within ourselves.

Kapha-type people tend to exhibit the qualities associated with the elements of that dosha—earth and water. They tend to be somewhat large-framed and heavy-set. Their skin is thick, cool, pale, and oily, and they prefer to live in warm climates. Kaphas tend to be earthy, stable people, with patient natures who like sharp and pungent foods. Kaphas learn very slowly, but they have a good long-term memory. They don't anger easily, but once a kapha is angry, he or she stays that way for a while. Kaphas sleep a lot and tend to be affectionate and emotionally secure.

The kapha elements are responsible for maintaining oiliness of the body and organs, general physical stability, virility, strength, and the fluidity of muscular and joint movement. When the kapha elements are out of balance, there are difficulties that arise within these functions, such as dryness or loss of oiliness, edema, emaciation, low immunity and susceptibility to disease, impotence, sterility, lethargy, confusion, and fatigue. The antidotes

Thyme helps energize kapha—earth and water elements. It has antiseptic properties that may help slow the aging process in vata, pitta, or kapha.

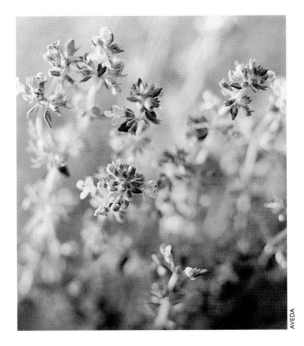

AVEDA

for illnesses stemming from kapha imbalances are things that have the opposite properties—those of fire and air.

The recommended diet for people with mainly kapha in their makeup is comprised largely of foods that are lighter. It includes apples, apricots, peaches, broccoli, cabbage, garlic, chilies, onions, okra, most peppers and spices, spinach, tomatoes, chicken, fish, and rice. Kaphas should avoid milk, cheese, avocado, bananas, dates, grapes, watermelon, cold food, cashew nuts, peanuts and almonds, especially during the winter season, when kapha is elevated in our environment.

Kapha types can benefit from vigorous exercise and should fight the inclination to be sedentary.

BALANCE

Ayurveda is a medical tradition aimed at balancing the body. It prescribes a variety of things for balancing the doshas and achieving good health. Among the tools it relies upon are six tastes that should be considered when you want to balance your body type. Those six tastes, or *rasas*, are sweet, sour, salty, bitter, pungent (spicy), and astringent (puckering). Each essential oil also has a primary dosha assigned to it and occasionally a secondary one.

After you've taken the questionnaire at the end of this chapter to determine your dominant doshas, you can use the following chart to understand how to use the six rasas to stay in balance. Also compare your dominant dosha to the list of oils that follows to identify the ones that will help your system stay in harmony.

BALANCING KAPHA

But life's a catch-22 when you're a pitta-kapha, because the kapha, or earth element, in me needs many of the things the pitta, or fire element in me, needs to avoid, like spicy foods. The kapha part of my nature also makes me resistant to exercise or movement of any kind. If I had it my way, I'd like to just sit around and get massaged all day. Three massages will do, as long as each lasts two-and-one-half hours. I'd like to have somebody move my body for me rather than have to exercise. Of course, if I lived this way, I'd be twice the size I am. I work to counteract this sedentary tendency of mine. And fortunately, my vata, or air element, is pretty active, too, and it keeps me from being content just to lounge all day.

THE SIX RASAS

| sweet | bitter | sour |
| pungent (spicy) | salty | astringent (puckering) |

The rasas are beneficial to the doshas as listed below

VATA Air		**PITTA** Fire		**KAPHA** Earth and Water	
Decreases	*Increases*	*Decreases*	*Increases*	*Decreases*	*Increases*
Salty	Pungent	Bitter	Pungent	Pungent	Sweet
Sour	Bitter	Astringent	Sour	Bitter	Sour
Sweet	Astringent	Sweet	Salty	Astringent	Salty

COMMON ESSENTIAL OILS AND THEIR AYURVEDIC DOSHAS

OIL NAME	PRIMARY KAPHA/PITTA/VATA	SECONDARY KAPHA/PITTA/VATA	OIL NAME	PRIMARY KAPHA/PITTA/VATA	SECONDARY KAPHA/PITTA/VATA
Ambrette seed oil	P	KV	Laurel leaf oil	V	
Amyris oil	K		Lavandin oil	V	
Anise oil, Chinese	K	V	Lavender, absolute green	V	P
Armoise oil	K		Lavender oil, pure	V	P
Basil oil, Commores	K		Lavender oil, spike	V	
Bay oil	V		Lemon oil, Star brand	V	P
Bergamot oil	V	K	Lemongrass oil	P	
Cajeput oil	V		Lime oil	P	VK
Camphor oil, white	V	P	Mandarin oil	V	
Cananga oil	P		Mandarin petitgrain	P	
Caraway seed oil	K		Marjoram oil, French	V	P
Cardamom oil	V	P	Marjoram oil, Spanish	V	K
Carrot seed oil	V		Melissa oil	P	
Cedarleaf oil	K		Menthe pouliot oil	V	P
Cedarwood oil	K	V	Mimosa, India	P	V
Celery seed oil	V		Myrrh oil	K	
Chamomile blue oil	V	K	Myrtle oil	K	
Chamomile oil	V	K	Narcissus	KV	
Chamomile oil, Roman	V		Neroli oil	P	
Cinnamon leaf oil	V	K	Nutmeg oil	V	
Cistus oil	V		Oakmoss	K	
Citronella java	V		Olibanum oil	P	K
Clary sage oil	K	V	Orange flower	K	
Clove bud oil	P	K	Orange oil, bitter	V	
Clove leaf oil	K	P	Orange oil, wild sweet	P	V
Copaiba oil	P		Orris	V	K
Coriander oil	V	PK	Palma rosa oil	V	
Cypress oil	V	P	Patchouli oil	V	
Cypriol oil	V		Pepper oil, black	K	V
Davanna essence	P		Peppermint oil	V	
Elemi oil	V		Petitgrain oil	P	
Estragon oil	V		Pimento berry oil	K	
Eucalyptus	V	K	Rose oil	P	
Fennel oil, sweet	K		Rosemary oil	V	
Galbanum oil	V		Sage oil	V	K
Genet absolute	K		Sandalwood oil	P	
Geranium oil	V	K	Spearmint oil	V	K
Ginger oil	K		Tangerine oil	V	
Grapefruit oil	V		Tea tree oil	K	
Guaiacwood oil	V	P	Thyme oil	V	
Hyssop oil	K		Violet leaves, absolute	P	
Jasmine	V	P	Wintergreen oil	V	
Juniper berry oil	V	P	Ylang-ylang	P	
Labdanum	K				

FOOD FACTS

Following is a guide to many common foods, their taste qualities, and their recommended amounts for each of the doshas, which comes from *A Simple Celebration* (Three Rivers Press, 1998) by Ginna Bell Bragg and David Simon, M.D.

BEVERAGES	TASTE	VATA	PITTA	KAPHA
Alcohol	pungent, sweet, bitter, sour	Some	Less	Less
Coffee	pungent, bitter	Less	Less	Some
Fruit juices				
Citrus	sweet, sour	More	Less	Less
Other	sweet, astringent	Less	More	More
Herbal teas				
Cinnamon, ginger, etc.	spicy	More	Less	More
Green, mint, etc.	astringent	Less	More	More
Milk and Dairy (see Dairy)				
Mineral water (carbonated)	bitter	Less	More	More
Soft drinks	sweet	Less	Less	Less
Tea (black, regular)	bitter, sweet, astringent	Less	More	More
Vegetable juices				
Carrot	sweet, astringent	More	Less	More
Cucumber	sweet, astringent	More	More	Less
Spinach	bitter, astringent	Less	Less	More

SWEETENERS	TASTE	VATA	PITTA	KAPHA
Honey	sweet	Some	More	More
Lactose—Milk, Sugar	sweet	Some	Some	Some
Malt, Rice, Barley syrup	sweet	More	More	Some
Maple syrup	sweet	More	More	More
Molasses	sweet	More	Less	Less
Raw sugar	sweet	More	More	Some
Rock candy	sweet	Some	Some	Some
Sucanat	sweet	Some	Some	Some
White sugar	sweet	Less	Less	Less

FLAVORINGS/ CONDIMENTS	TASTE	VATA	PITTA	KAPHA
Bragg's Liquid Aminos	astringent, salty	Some	Less	Less
Carob	sweet, astringent	Some	More	More
Chocolate	pungent, bitter	Some	Less	Less
Cornstarch	sweet	Some	Some	Some
Mayonnaise	sour, sweet	Some	Less	Less
Mustard	pungent	More	Less	More
Salt	salty	Some	Less	Less
Vegit	all	Some	Some	Some
Vinegar	sour	Some	Less	Less

MEAT AND FISH	TASTE	VATA	PITTA	KAPHA
Beef	sweet	Some	Less	Less
Chicken, Turkey	sweet	Some	Some	Some
Duck	sweet	More	Less	Less
Lamb	sweet	Some	Less	Less

MEAT AND FISH	TASTE	VATA	PITTA	KAPHA
Pork	sweet	Less	Less	Less
Venison	sweet	More	Less	Less
Fish	sweet, salty	More	Some	Less
Shellfish	sweet	More	Less	Less
Animal oils				
Eggs	sweet	More	Less	Less
Lard	sweet	Some	Some	Less

OILS	TASTE	VATA	PITTA	KAPHA
Almond	sweet, bitter	More	Less	Less
Avocado	sweet, astringent	More	Some	Less
Canola	sweet	Less	Some	More
Corn	sweet	Less	Some	Some
Coconut	sweet	Some	More	Less
Flaxseed/Linseed	pungent, sweet	More	Less	More
Margarine	sweet	Less	Some	Some
Mustard	pungent	Some	Less	More
Olive	sweet	More	Some	Less
Peanut	sweet	Some	Less	Some
Safflower	sweet, pungent	More	Some	More
Sesame	sweet	More	Less	Less
Soy	sweet, astringent	Some	Some	Some
Sunflower	sweet	Some	Some	More

BEANS, LEGUMES	TASTE	VATA	PITTA	KAPHA
Aduki beans	sweet, astringent	Some	More	More
Black gram (Indian)	sweet, astringent	Less	More	Some
Fava beans	sweet, astringent	Less	More	More
Chickpeas	sweet, astringent	Some	Some	Less
Kidney beans	sweet, astringent	Some	Some	Some
Lentils	sweet, astringent	Less	Some	More
Lima beans	sweet, astringent	Some	More	More
Mung beans	sweet, astringent	More	More	Some
Peanuts	sweet, astringent	Less	Less	Some
Pinto beans	sweet, astringent	Less	Some	Some
Soybeans	sweet, astringent	Less	Some	More
Tofu	sweet, astringent	Some	More	Some
Split peas	sweet, astringent	Less	Some	Some

DAIRY	TASTE	VATA	PITTA	KAPHA
Butter	sweet	More	More	Less
Buttermilk	sour, astringent	More	Less	Some
Cheese	sweet	Some	Some	Less
Cottage cheese	sweet	More	More	Less
Cream	sweet	More	More	Less
Ghee	sweet	More	More	Some
Ice cream	sweet	Less	Less	Less
Kefir	sour	More	Some	Some
Milk	sweet	More	More	Less
Paneer cheese	sweet, sour	Some	Some	Some
Sour cream	sweet, sour	More	Less	Less
Yogurt	sweet, sour	Less	Less	Less

FRUITS	TASTE	VATA	PITTA	KAPHA
Apples	sweet, astringent	Some	More	More
Apricots	sweet, sour	Some	Less	Some
Avocados	sweet	More	Some	Less
Bananas	sweet, astringent	Some	Less	Less
Blueberries	sweet, astringent	More	More	Less
Cranberries	astringent, sweet	Less	More	More
Cherries	sweet, sour	More	Less	Less
Dates	sweet	More	More	Less
Figs	sweet, astringent	More	More	Less
Grapefruits	sour	More	Some	More
Grapes	sweet, sour	More	More	Less
Lemons	sour, astringent	More	Less	Less
Lemon, Orange zest	bitter	Less	More	More
Limes	sour	More	Less	Less
Mangoes	sweet, sour	More	Some	Less
Melons	sweet	Less	More	Less
Nectarines	sweet, sour	More	Some	Less
Oranges	sweet, sour	Some	Some	Less
Papayas	sweet	More	Some	Some
Peaches	sweet, sour	Some	Less	Less
Pears	sweet	Some	More	Some
Persimmons	sweet, astringent	Some	More	Less
Pineapples	sweet, sour	More	More	Less
Plums	sweet, sour	Some	Some	Less
Prunes	sweet, sour	More	More	Some
Pomegranates	sweet, astringent, sour	Some	More	Some
Raisins, Currants	sweet	Less	Some	More
Raspberries, Blackberries	sweet, sour	More	Some	Less
Strawberries	sweet, sour, astringent	More	More	Less
Tangerines	sour, sweet	Some	Less	Some

HERBS, SPICES	TASTE	VATA	PITTA	KAPHA
Allspice	pungent	More	Less	More
Anise	pungent	Less	Less	More
Asafoetida (hing)	pungent	More	Less	More
Basil	pungent	More	Some	More
Bay leaves	pungent	More	Less	More
Black pepper	pungent	Some	Less	More
Calamus	pungent	More	Less	More
Caraway	pungent	More	Some	More
Cardamom	pungent, sweet	More	Some	More
Catnip	pungent	Some	Some	Some
Cayenne	pungent	Some	Less	More
Chamomile	pungent, bitter	More	More	More
Cinnamon	pungent, bitter	More	Some	More
Cloves	pungent	More	Some	More
Coriander	pungent, bitter	More	More	More
Cumin	pungent	More	Some	More
Dill	pungent	Some	Some	Some
Fennel	pungent	More	More	Some
Fenugreek	bitter	More	Less	More
Garlic	all but sour	More	Less	More
Ginger	pungent, sweet	More	Less	More

HERBS, SPICES	TASTE	VATA	PITTA	KAPHA
Horseradish	pungent	Some	Less	More
Hyssop	pungent, astringent	More	Less	More
Italian seasoning	pungent	More	Less	More
Lemon verbena	pungent, sour	Some	Some	Some
Lemongrass	pungent, sour	Some	Some	Some
Marjoram	pungent	More	Less	More
Mint	pungent	Some	Some	Some
Mustard	pungent	Some	Less	More
Nutmeg	pungent, astringent	More	Some	Some
Oregano	pungent	More	Less	More
Paprika	pungent	Some	Some	Some
Peppermint	pungent	Some	Some	Some
Poppy seeds	pungent, astringent, sweet	More	Less	More
Rosemary	pungent, bitter	More	Some	More
Saffron	pungent	Some	Some	Some
Sage	pungent, astringent	More	Less	More
Spearmint	pungent	Some	Some	Some
Star anise	pungent, sweet	More	Less	More
Tarragon	pungent	More	Less	More
Thyme	pungent	More	Less	More
Turmeric	bitter, pungent, astringent	Some	Some	More

NUTS, SEEDS	TASTE	VATA	PITTA	KAPHA
Almonds	sweet, bitter	More	Less	Less
Brazil nuts	sweet	More	Less	Less
Cashews	sweet	More	Less	Less
Coconut	sweet	Some	More	Some
Filberts	sweet	More	Less	Less
Lotus seeds	sweet, astringent	Less	More	Less
Macadamia nuts	sweet	More	Less	Less
Mustard seeds	pungent	More	Less	More
Pecans	sweet, bitter	More	Less	Less
Pine nuts (piñon)	sweet	More	Some	Less
Pistachios	sweet	More	Less	Less
Pumpkin seeds	sweet	Some	Some	Some
Sesame seeds	sweet	More	Some	Some
Sunflower seeds	sweet, bitter	Some	More	Some
Walnuts	sweet	More	Less	Less

VEGETABLES	TASTE	VATA	PITTA	KAPHA
Artichokes	sweet, astringent	Less	More	Some
Asparagus	sweet, bitter, astringent	Some	More	More
Bean sprouts	astringent, sweet	Less	More	More
Beans (green)	sweet, astringent	Less	More	More
Beets	bitter, sweet	More	Some	More
Bell peppers	sweet, astringent	Less	Some	Some
Broccoli	bitter, astringent	Less	More	More
Brussels sprouts	astringent, sweet	Less	More	More
Cabbage	astringent, sweet	Less	More	More
Carrots	sweet, pungent	More	Some	More

		VATA	PITTA	KAPHA
Cauliflower	sweet, astringent	Some	More	Some
Celery	bitter, astringent	Some	More	More
Chilis (hot pepper)	pungent	More	Less	More
Cilantro	pungent	More	More	More
Corn	sweet	Less	Some	Some
Cucumbers	sweet, astringent	Some	More	Less
Eggplants	bitter	Some	Some	Some
Fennel	pungent	More	Less	More
Jerusalem artichokes	sweet	More	More	Less
Jicama	sweet	More	More	Less
Lettuce	bitter, astringent	Less	More	More
Mushrooms	sweet, astringent	Less	More	More
Mustard greens	pungent, bitter	More	Less	More
Okra	sweet	More	More	Some
Onions, cooked (leeks, scallions, chives, shallots)	sweet, pungent	Some	Some	More
Onions, raw (leeks, scallions, chives, shallots)	sweet, pungent	Less	Less	Less
Parsley	pungent, astringent	More	Some	Some
Peas (green or snow)	sweet, astringent	Less	More	More
Potatoes	astringent	Less	Some	Some
Radishes	bitter	More	Some	More
Seaweed	salty, astringent	More	Some	Some
Spinach (chard)	bitter	Some	Some	Some
Squash				
Acorn	sweet	Less	Some	Some
Winter	sweet	Less	Some	Less
Zucchini, Yellow Crookneck	sweet	Less	More	Less
Sweet potatoes	sweet	More	Some	Less
Tomatoes	sweet, sour	Less	Some	Some
Turnips/Rutabagas	astringent	Less	Some	More

GRAINS	TASTE	VATA	PITTA	KAPHA
Barley	sweet	Some	More	More
Buckwheat	sweet	Some	Some	Some
Corn	sweet	Some	Some	Some
Couscous	sweet, astringent	Less	More	Less
Granola				
Dried grains	sweet, astringent	Less	Some	More
Millet	sweet	Some	Some	Some
Oats	sweet	More	More	Less
Quinoa	sweet, astringent	Some	Some	More
Rice				
Basmati	sweet	More	More	Some
Brown	sweet	More	Some	Less
Refined, White	sweet	Some	Some	Less
Rye	sweet, astringent	Less	Some	Some
Spelt	sweet, astringent	More	More	Some
White flour	sweet, astringent	Less	Less	Less
Whole wheat flour	sweet, astringent	More	More	Less

AYURVEDA AND EATING

	VATA *Air*	PITTA *Fire*	KAPHA *Earth and Water*
Symptoms	Restlessness Listless sleep Anxiety Exhaustion Weight loss	Rashes Irritability Temper Hair loss or graying	Allergies Sluggishness Oversleeping Weight gain
Foods to enjoy	Warm, oily foods Sweet, salty, sour Wheat Oats White rice Dairy Oils Sweet fruits Well-cooked vegetables Nuts Poultry Seafood	Cool foods Bitter, sweet Rice Wheat Milk and butter Olive, sunflower oils Sweet fruits Green vegetables Poultry Egg whites	Light, dry, warm foods Barley, corn, rye Milk Honey Apples Pears Beans Poultry
Foods to skip	Dry, cold, strong, bitter foods Yogurt, cheese Dried fruit Raw vegetables Beans Beef	Hot, sour, salty foods Spicy Wheat Corn, sesame oil Sour foods Acidic vegetables (garlic, onions) Peanuts Sesame seeds Beef Seafood Egg yolks	Oily, cold foods Rice Cheese Yogurt Sweet fruits Salt Nuts Tomatoes Cucumbers Zucchini Beef Seafood Pork

Once you've completed the questionnaire at the end of this chapter, use the chart below to better understand which foods will help you overcome certain common ailments.

Although we possess characteristics of all the elements and of each of the doshas, most of us are influenced most strongly by two of the element combinations. Using the questionnaire and the analyses that go along with

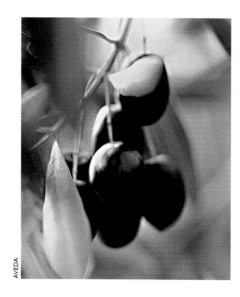

AVEDA

O*live oil can be enjoyed by those of all doshas, though it benefits vata most.*

it, you can determine for yourself what your makeup is. That will help you make decisions about the details of your nurturing daily routines as you go along through the chapters ahead.

If you'd like to get professional help diagnosing your dominant doshas and identifying imbalances, you can seek the attention of doctors trained in the Ayurvedic tradition. Some of the better-known M.D.'s who incorporate Ayurveda into their practices are Dr. Scott Gerson, Dr. Deepak Chopra, Dr. Carrie Demers, and Dr. David Simon—all of whom have written great books on Ayurvedic medicine, which can be helpful, too. To find doctors and other practitioners of Ayurvedic medicine in your community, talk to your regular doctor, or check with the local health food store to see if the people who run it might know of any.

If you have the time and money, you can go to the Himalayan Ayurvedic Center, a hospital in India overlooking the snow peaks of the Himalayas, which has a five-day retreat program for evaluating people's doshas and coaching them in a customized, healthy set of daily rituals—just like the ones you'll find in this book.

YOUR AYURVEDIC MAKEUP

The following questionnaire will help you to determine your dominant doshas. Just answer all the questions in the vata, pitta, and kapha sections, and then add up your score for each dosha. Very simply, the dosha for which you have the highest score is your dominant one. You may have similar scores for two, which means you are dominant in both.

AYURVEDA QUESTIONNAIRE

VATA ELEMENT

	not at all	slightly	somewhat	moderately	very
▶ I tend to think and act quickly.	1	2	3	(4)	5
▶ I am lively and enthusiastic by nature.	1	2	3	(4)	5
▶ I tend to be thin and rarely gain weight.	1	2	(3)	4	5
▶ My daily schedule of eating meals, going to sleep, and awakening tends to vary from day to day.	1	2	3	4	(5)
▶ Under stress, I tend to worry and become anxious.	1	2	(3)	4	5
▶ I speak quickly and am a lively conversationalist.	1	2	3	(4)	5
▶ My feet and hands tend to be cool.	1	2	(3)	4	5
▶ I tend to have difficulty falling asleep or awaken easily.	(1)	2	3	4	5
▶ My digestion tends to be irregular with frequent gas or bloating.	1	2	3	4	(5)
▶ I tend to eat quickly, finishing my meals before others at my table.	1	2	3	(4)	5

Total for vata (air) section: __36__

Healthy, balanced vata element constitutions are flexible, creative, dynamic, enthusiastic, and energetic.

PITTA ELEMENT

	not at all	slightly	somewhat	moderately	very
▶ My skin is sensitive, sunburns, or breaks out easily.	1	2	3	4	(5)
▶ I have a tendency toward indigestion or heartburn.	1	2	3	4	(5)
▶ I tend to be a perfectionist with a low tolerance for errors.	1	2	(3)	4	5
▶ I commonly have more than one bowel movement per day.	1	2	(3)	4	5
▶ I feel rested with less than eight hours of sleep.	1	(2)	3	4	5

	not at all	slightly	somewhat	moderately	very
▸ I think critically, am a good debater, and can argue a point forcefully.	1	2	3	4	⑤
▸ When pressured, I tend to become irritable or impatient.	1	2	③	4	5
▸ If I begin a new project, I tend not to stop until I've completed it.	1	2	③	4	5
▸ I have a strong appetite and can eat large quantities of food if I choose.	1	2	③	4	5
▸ I tend to perform my activities with precision and orderliness.	1	2	③	4	5

Total for pitta (fire) section: _____35_____

Healthy, balanced pitta element constitutions show warmth, skill, leadership, intelligence, and compassion.

KAPHA ELEMENT

	not at all	slightly	somewhat	moderately	very
▸ I am a good listener. I speak only when I feel I have something important to say.	1	②	3	4	5
▸ I have a tendency toward chronic sinus congestion, asthma, or excessive phlegm.	1	2	3	④	5
▸ I have slow digestion and tend to feel heavy after eating.	1	2	③	4	5
▸ I tend to eat slowly.	1	②	3	4	5
▸ My skin is usually soft and smooth.	①	2	3	4	5
▸ I tend to perform activities in a slow-paced manner.	1	②	3	4	5
▸ I tend to be loyal and devoted in my relationships.	1	2	3	4	⑤
▸ I tend to gain weight easily and have difficulty losing extra pounds.	1	2	③	4	5
▸ I tend to be steady and methodical with consistent energy and endurance.	①	2	3	4	5
▸ I tend to be calm by nature and seldom lose my temper.	①	2	3	4	5

Total for kapha (water) section: _____24_____

Healthy, balanced kapha element constitutions exhibit strength, endurance, stability, calm, and contentment.

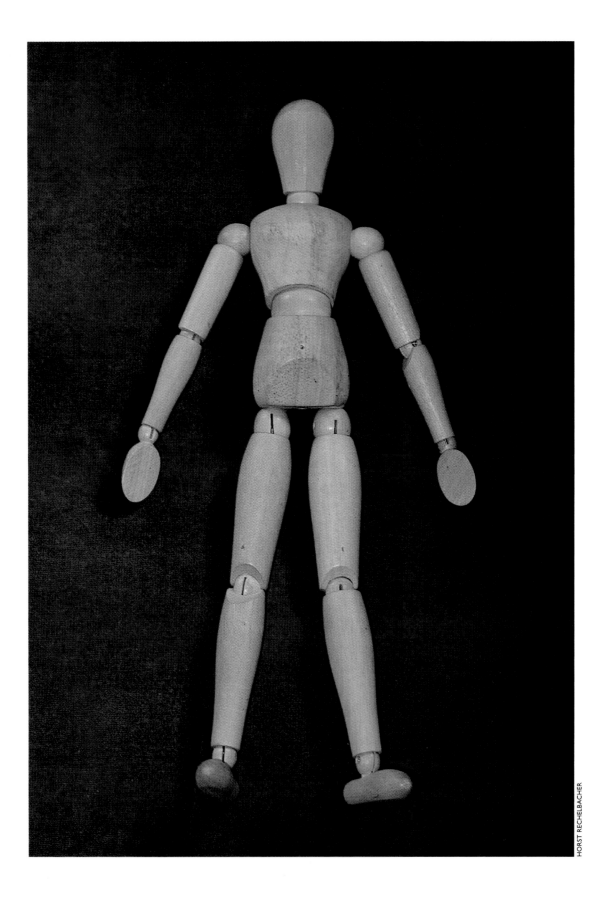

4

Good Vibrations

The Chakras or Vibrational Zones

To live life is not merely to breathe, it is to act; it is to make use of our organs, senses, faculties, of all those parts of ourselves which give us the feeling of existence.

—JEAN-JACQUES ROUSSEAU

EVERY ONE OF US IS AFFECTED BY THE FIVE ELEMENTS, earth, air, water, fire, and space. As we learned in the last chapter, we are all influenced more by some of the elements than others. In this chapter, I'll discuss the centers in our bodies where each of the elements makes its headquarters and how the energy vibrations within those vortexes direct our various body functions and systems. In the Ayurvedic tradition of medicine, these centers are called *chakras*, and there are seven of them. Other ancient and indigenous traditions recognize these centers, too, but by different names. The chakras are vibrational zones in our bodies that carry information about all our organs and our emotions as they affect our physiology.

It is through these vibrational zones that the life-force energy—known in the Indian tradition as *prana*, and in Chinese tradition as *chi*—flows to the rest of the body. We are filled with and surrounded by this life-force energy. The chakra system is a way of understanding how we tap into that energy pool and the biological aspect of it in our bodies.

Later in the book, I'll discuss the concept of reflexology, and how the chakras and their functions affect and are affected by different zones on our feet. The bottoms of our feet are actually road maps of our energy zones and the rest of our bodies; they can tell us a lot about the condition of its various parts and systems. We can work toward healing ourselves through specific techniques in foot massage, called reflexology, which I'll discuss in greater detail in the chapter on massage.

There is a lot we can understand about our bodies, minds, and spirits once we understand how our chakras operate. By knowing how they function and what systems they govern—and how they pertain to our own elemental makeups—we can take further steps toward tailoring a set of healthy nurturing daily practices.

Balancing the flow of energy through our chakras is part of the formula for bringing our bodies, minds, and spirits into the zone of bliss. Once we know what each of the chakras is responsible for, and how they affect the rest of our bodies, we can take what I call a "chakra inventory," and figure out how to bring those different chakras into balance. From there, we are better able to ground ourselves, through controlled breathing, meditation, and a regimen of other nurturing practices. It works the other way around, too. Through meditation and other grounding practices, we can work toward putting our chakras into balance. Just as with everything else within our lives, we have a symbiotic relationship with these energy centers and can influence how they operate and affect our lives.

The seven chakra zones are aligned vertically, from the base of our spine to the top of our head, but they affect more than just the localized body regions where they sit. Rather, each of them governs different, larger sectors of our beings. On another level, six of the seven energy centers also correspond with a different element, and five of them with a sensory perception. They are all associated with a color and a level of consciousness.

Over time, we can each work through the chakras to a state of maximum consciousness. This takes years of learning and practice, but there is the opportunity for mastery at each level. We can take a daily chakra inventory and set new goals each day. When we put our intention behind our energy, we are better able to reach those goals and to work through any fear, anger, guilt, and addictions we might have.

THE ZONING BOARD

The following is a basic guide to understanding the seven chakras of the human body, how they affect our systems and behavior, as well as how our systems and behavior affect them. The color associated with each of the chakras can be used as an added tool in meditation when we are interested in addressing issues of that zone. For example, if you're dealing with issues that stem from the pleasure center, or chakra 2, you might meditate on its color, red. Let's take a closer look.

Chakra 1—The Root Center

This is the vibrational zone of stability, survival, and safety, and the chakra through which we can become grounded. We are all electromagnetic matter. There is a cosmic interactive dance taking place within us and around us continually. Chakra 1, the root center, is the zone through which we may get into a state of low vibration and groundedness in relation to the energy fields we move through daily.

The root center is located at the base of the spine, and it is symbolized by one downward triangle. Appropriately, the element associated with this chakra is earth. The sensory perception it governs is smell. The color assigned to it is a subtle bluish red.

This chakra rules issues of basic existence and survival, such as our animal instinct of "eat or be eaten."

The physical regions that the root center oversees are the reproductive organs in women, the prostate in men, feet to knees, the back of legs, the hips and thighs, the veins and arteries in our lower limbs, the hamstrings, and the lower colon. Fittingly, these are the physical portions of our bodies that determine our ability to stand firm. The functions that the root center oversees are solidity, stability, groundedness, and body-consciousness.

When the root center is in balance, we feel secure and brave. When we experience feelings of fear, tension, and selfishness; varicose veins or phlebitis, it is often an indication that our root center is out of balance.

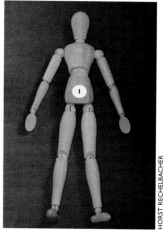

HORST RECHELBACHER

Element: Earth
Perception: Smell
Color: Yellow

SYMPTOMS OF IMBALANCE	ULTIMATE BALANCE
Fear	Security
Tension	Balance
Selfishness	

Chakra 2—The Pleasure Center

The pleasure center is the source of all desire and addictions, and the quest for satisfaction within our bodies. This is the chakra that is the center for all of our attachments—to people, food, substances, and behaviors. On a grander scale, whereas chakra 1 is concerned with the survival of the individual, chakra 2 is concerned with the survival of the species at large. This perpetuation can be guaranteed only when people are stimulated to seek pleasure, particularly sexual pleasure. This is the vibrational zone that ensures that will happen.

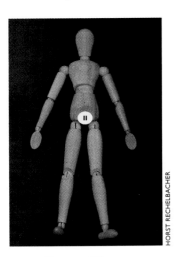

Element: Water
Perception: Taste

SYMPTOMS OF IMBALANCE	ULTIMATE BALANCE
Addictions	Satisfaction
Fear of Aging	Contentment with Self
	Faithfulness

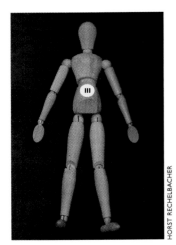

Element: Fire
Perception: Eyesight

SYMPTOMS OF IMBALANCE	ULTIMATE BALANCE
Anger	Patience
Laziness	Energy
Insomnia	Assertiveness
	Confidence

Also fittingly, the pleasure center is the vibrational zone that is responsible for sensuality and beauty, the bait in the hunt for sexual satisfaction and propagation.

The pleasure center is located, appropriately, near the prostate gland in men, and near the reproductive organs in women. Its symbol is two triangles, one upward, one downward—the symbols for male and female reproductive systems—touching at their bases, forming a diamond. The element associated with it is water; the perception, taste; and the color, a purplish red.

While the pleasure center does govern sexual desire, that isn't the only appetite it controls. This is also the seat of hunger and thirst, for food, alcohol, and conquest.

The physical regions governed by the pleasure center are the female reproductive organs, the male prostate, the pelvis, the front of legs, the quadriceps, the intestines, and the lower back. The functions it controls are hormone secretion and libido.

When our pleasure center is in balance, we feel satisfied, content within ourselves, and we tend to be faithful. When we have addictions, fear of aging, dissatisfaction, hatred, a lack of discipline, or infidelity, it is often a sign that our pleasure center is out of balance.

Chakra 3—The Energy Center

While all the chakras conduct energy in some form, this chakra conducts that brand of energy which relates to activity, strength, and physical power, as well as emotional fortitude. This is the vibrational zone that is in charge of distributing energy to all other parts of the body. It is symbolized by an upward triangle.

Chakra 3, or the energy center, located in the solar plexus, has fire as its element, eyesight as its perception, and fiery orange-red as its color.

In addition to sending energy throughout the body, the energy center is responsible for digestion and inner cleansing, strength, personal power, aggression, ego, and identity.

The physical regions influenced by the energy center are the abdomen, the area behind the stomach, the pancreas, the spleen, the adrenal glands, the upper colon, the kidneys, the liver, and the area above the navel. The functions of chakra 3 are burning fuel, digesting food, and regulating chakras 1 and 2.

We are patient, energetic, assertive, and confident when our energy center is balanced. When our energy center is not well balanced, we might feel angry, lazy, impatient, have a lack of confidence, suffer insomnia, or have a tendency to procrastinate.

Chakra 4—The Heart Center

All the love songs and imagery that refer to the heart as the center of all emotional activity are right on the mark. While to some extent, most emotions pass through the brain, their energy vibration is processed in chakra 4, the heart center, located smack dab between the breasts, near the cardiac muscle.

The perception associated with the heart center is, fittingly, touch. The element is air, the color a green-yellow with some warm maroon tinges, and the symbol is two triangles intertwined to form a star.

This vibrational zone handles our emotional energy and enables us to feel, emotionally and physically. It also acts as an integrating center for the yin and yang, male and female, of the upper and lower body regions.

The physical areas that the heart center oversees include the chest, the lungs, the heart, the lymphatic system, the breasts, and the interior area above the diaphragm. The functions it rules are breathing, nurturing, purification of the blood, lymphatic flow, loving, and compassion.

When our heart center is in balance, we feel compassionate, responsible, nurturing, open to humor, lighthearted, and in harmony with ourselves and others. When our heart center is out of balance, we may act ungrateful, greedy, insensitive to others, abusive, overly talkative, and we may suffer poor circulation.

Chakra 5—The Throat Center

When humans express themselves, they do so most often through the sound of verbal communication, which originates in the throat. It seems right, then, that the throat center, chakra 5, is the source of that which we express—all creative processes originate here.

Symbolized by a diamond, the throat chakra is located in the pharynx, or throat. Its sensory perception is hearing; its element is space, or ether; its color is a bluish white.

The throat chakra governs the hollow of the neck, the throat, the ears, the thymus, the salivary glands, the tongue, the teeth, and the lymphatic nodes in the neck. Its functions are expression in general, talking specifically, and motivating the creative process.

When our throat center is in balance, we experience the ability to trust,

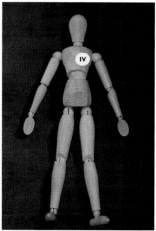

HORST RECHELBACHER

Element: Air
Perception: Touch

SYMPTOMS OF IMBALANCE	ULTIMATE BALANCE
Ungrateful	Compassionate
Hasty	Responsible
Talkative	Nurturing
Poor Circulation	

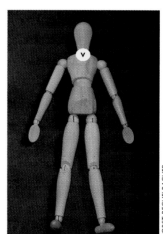

HORST RECHELBACHER

Element: Ether, Space
Perception: Hearing

SYMPTOMS OF IMBALANCE	ULTIMATE BALANCE
Has Romantic Crushes	Trusting
Prone to Idolatry	Devoted
Has Creative Block	Creative
Suffers from Rejection	Accepting

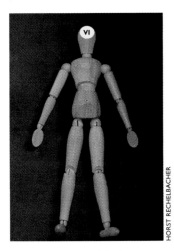

Element: Mind
Color: White

SYMPTOMS OF IMBALANCE	ULTIMATE BALANCE
Meanness	Wise
Lack of Discrimination	Knowing
Lack of Awareness	Discriminating

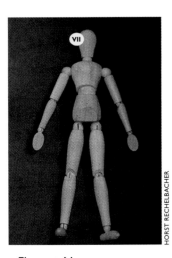

Element: None
Color: White, bluish purple

SYMPTOMS OF IMBALANCE	ULTIMATE BALANCE
Ignorance	Spiritual Consciousness
	Awareness of the Interconnectiveness of All Things

devotion, creativity, and acceptance. When our throat center is out of balance, we are likely to form romantic crushes, idolize people, feel rejected or paranoid, and experience creative blocks.

Chakra 6—The Eyebrow Center

Naturally this chakra, which is in charge of intellect, is located where it seems it should be, right in the center of the forehead. More precisely, the eyebrow center is located on the nasociliary nerve. The eyebrow center, or chakra 6, takes care of all things intuitive and intellectual. It is also responsible for our conscious awareness; so, in our efforts to become more conscious through our daily rituals, we will want to become very familiar with this vibrational zone.

The element associated with it is space, its color is blue-white, and it is symbolized by an upward triangle contained in a circle.

The eyebrow center is responsible for the following physical areas: the head, forehead, eyebrows, the brain, the hypothalamus, the limbic system, the eyes, the medulla oblongata, and the pituitary gland. The functions it oversees are rectifying faults in other centers, understanding, intuition, awareness, cognitive intellect, involuntary body functions, and sensitivity to light.

When the eyebrow center is in balance, we are wise, knowledgeable, and discriminating. When the eyebrow center is out of balance, we might be absentminded, mean, unaware, indiscriminate, suffer from Alzheimer's disease, or be egotistical and narrow-minded.

Chakra 7—The Crown Center

At the top of the head sits the crown center. This is the vibrational zone that is responsible for our cosmic consciousness. It is in this chakra that our awareness of our relationship to all beings and things in the universe is controlled.

The colors associated with this vibrational zone are white and a radiant, iridescent white, and it is symbolized by a full spectrum diamond shape, known in India as the lotus with a thousand petals.

The physical areas ruled by the crown center are the top of the head and the area above the head. Its functions are self-realization, spirituality, and universal consciousness.

When our crown center is in balance, we are spiritually conscious and aware of the full spectrum of all things in the universe and their interconnectedness. When our crown center is out of balance, we might be ignorant and psychically out of tune with ourselves and everything around us.

SIMPLE REFLEX

A third diagnostic and healing method, reflexology, can be used in conjunction with attention to our elemental makeups and awareness of our chakras and the more than 360 energy substations or meridian points located between the chakras on our bodies. Reflexology teaches that organs and glands correspond with different areas of the soles of the feet. We can stimulate these glands and organs by stimulating the corresponding foot areas. And, we can examine the feet to look for clues regarding what might be happening in the rest of our bodies.

In the second half the of the book, in the chapter on massage, I'll provide more details on reflexology and how to perform it on yourself and others.

Now that we know how to use the diagnostic tools of Ayurveda, the chakras, and reflexology, we can move on to the second half of the book. There, I'll help you tailor your own individual daily routine of nurturing practices, using what you've learned about yourself so far.

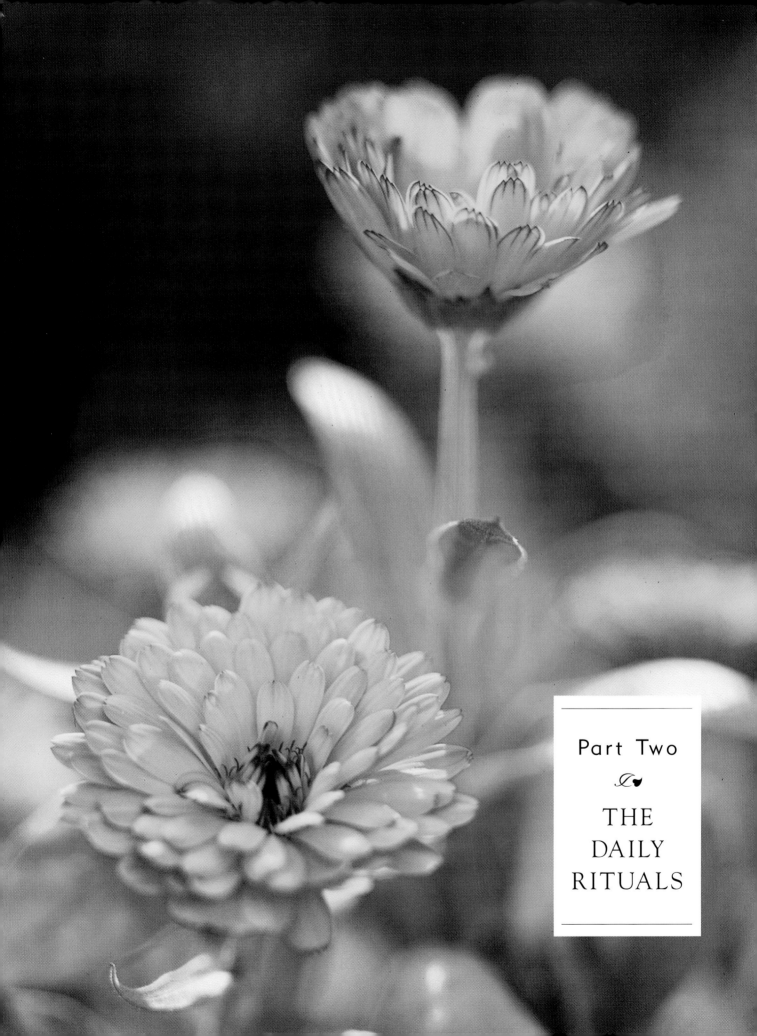

Part Two

𝓛❧

THE
DAILY
RITUALS

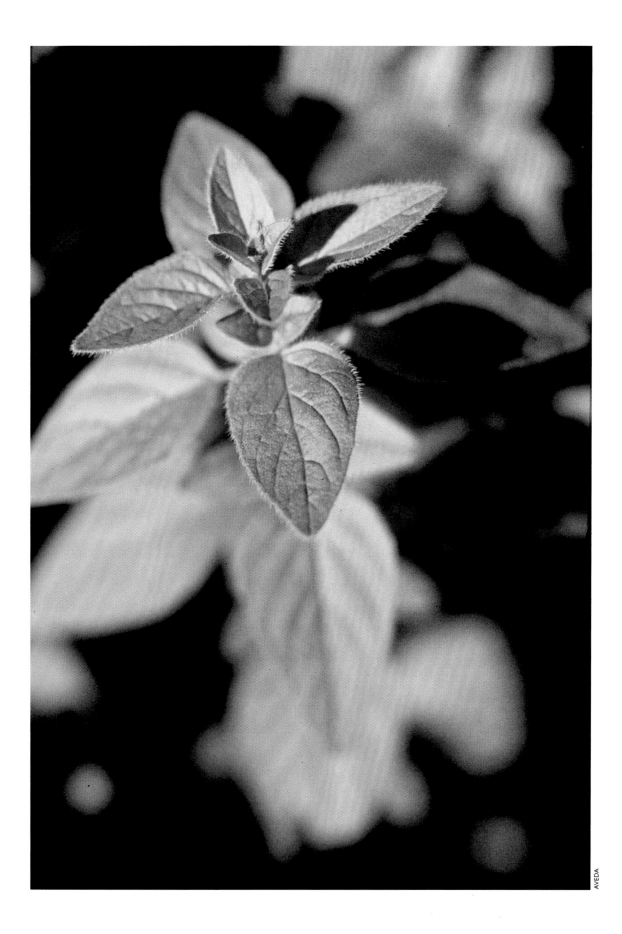

5

A Day in the Life

A Sample Day of Practices

Life does not need to be changed. Only our intents and actions do.

—SWAMI RAMA

NOW THAT WE HAVE TAKEN A LOOK AT THE BENEFITS of a daily routine of nurturing habits, and we've had a chance to learn a bit about our own constitutions, it's time to concentrate on the individual physical, mental, and spiritual practices that might constitute our daily rituals.

In this chapter, I'll outline my own personal preferences for a daily routine. My recommendations take into consideration what I have learned that benefits my own constitution through years of study around the world.

In the chapters that follow, I'll go into each of the rituals I mention here more deeply, and lay out some options for personalization within those practices. These variations on body movement, foods, essential oils, and herbs, minerals, etc., will take into account the differences you might have in dosha or just help open your mind to the wide choice of possibilities you can select from when creating your regimen.

As I've said before, we are all very similar but very different at the same time. We each will benefit the most from a specialized set of nurturing practices, informed by our likes and dislikes and our elemental makeups. We can make specific choices about which rituals work best for us, and which plant essences, foods, scents, oils, shampoos, conditioners, fixatives, and other cosmetics suit us individually. You can make those choices as you go along through each chapter ahead. I want to share with you here what I have done.

THE ORDER OF THINGS

Here's a brief synopsis of a good daily routine, which is based on the way that I conduct "my business of being" on most days. Later, I'll go into each of the times of day, and the routines suggested for them, in greater detail. You will see immediately, however, that the morning is the most ritual-intensive section of my routine. I suggest that you fashion your day similarly. Consciously preparing our minds, bodies, and spirits for the day changes our experience of what follows dramatically. Focusing on each part of ourselves before the busy day begins puts our goals into perspective, relaxes our bodies, makes our spirits receptive and our minds open. Destressed and targeted, we perform our best. We need to get up earlier to make time for all the things that help us to be conscious and content in every moment.

Morning

SACRED SILENCE

When you wake up in the morning, what is the first thing that you do? Do you roll over and go back to sleep or bound out of bed on the run? Either way, there is an important step you are missing. A moment or two can change the whole tenor of your day. Before we do anything, before we even get out of bed, there is something we should all do: Create a mental space for ourselves, and use that space to think about why we are here, and to continue the affirmations we made the night before. Realize that we are here, on this Earth, in this life, for a good reason. Make a point to be happy to be here—before you engage in even the smallest activity. The first thought of the day should be positive and special. That, for me, is the first ritual of the day.

BLOSSOM BREATH

Next comes what is probably a very common first ritual for many people already—cleaning the mouth. This is a good thing to do right after getting out of bed, because we want to get all of the toxins out of the mouth as soon as possible. We want to brush our teeth and floss. Tongue scraping is also a very beneficial habit that removes the many toxins that accumulate on the tongue through the night. I use a tongue scraper, but a spoon will also do the trick. Simply scrape, then spit.

MINIMASSAGE

Now it's time to start working our bodies. It begins, for me, with an all-over scalp and body massage. I start with either jojoba oil, sesame oil, or AVEDA Adaptive Massage Base with jojoba and plant triglicerides, such as clarified coconut oil. To my massage oil base, I add other essential oils. I often add an energizing plant or flower essence, like peppermint, in with the oil to stimulate my skin and senses. But be careful: Essential oils need to be used in very small concentrations or they can burn the skin. Never put essential oils on the skin without first mixing them into an oil base. Be sure to ask a knowledgeable salesperson at the health food store or herb shop where you buy your essential oils to recommend a safe essential-oil-to-massage-oil ratio. AVEDA has lots of premixed massage oils that have safe essence concentration levels. Sample them in any AVEDA concept shop and choose the ones you love.

My five- or ten-minute massage is a great way to get my blood flowing and promote healthy lymphatic drainage. I start at my head, then move to my face, neck, chest, arms, and so forth all the way down my body to the bottoms of my feet. I also use this as a time for self-examination. Through this practice I have come to know every inch of myself and, therefore, am immediately aware if something is amiss. Knowledge of our own bodies is very important to our health, inner-balance, and overall well-being.

GOOD-MORNING MOVEMENT

Movement is next on the agenda. Having warmed up my muscles and circulatory system with a self-massage, at this stage I am ready to engage in either energizing or calming exercise—or both. Some people like do some breathing, yoga postures, and some stretches or some tai chi positions before moving into a more vigorous form of motion, such as aerobic activity. This is a good time of the day for aerobic exercises, like running, swimming, cycling, and using cardiovascular machines such as a treadmill, cross-country skier, or step machine.

Being dominated partly by the kapha dosha, or earth element, my inclination is to exercise almost never. I like to sit around. But I know that movement is key to a healthy mind, body, and spirit, so I fight this tendency. Most mornings, I begin my movement routine with some deep bellows breathing, followed by a series of gentle yoga postures known collectively as

TOO MUCH OF A GOOD THING . . .

Certain essential oils are highly volatile substances that can be toxic and burn your skin if they're used in too high a concentration with a base oil. These should be highly diluted, consisting of less than 1 percent in a mixture with a base oil, and never taken orally except when under the direction of a medical doctor who has been practicing with essential oils for a long time. Pregnant women should avoid them altogether. Before using any of the following oils, find out the right essence-to-base-oil ratio from an herbalist, a doctor who practices with oils, or a knowledgeable salesperson:

- anise seed
- bitter almond
- bitter fennel
- camphor (brown and yellow)
- cinnamon
- clary sage
- clove (leaf, stem, and bulb)
- hyssop
- juniper
- myrrh
- pennyroyal
- pine
- sage
- savory
- wormwood
- wintergreen

the sun salutation. These postures awaken all the body systems, tone the muscles, and also provide the inversion necessary to create balance in all areas of the body. I hold the yoga postures for different lengths of time each day, depending on my mood and how my body feels. It is important not to be too rigid with yourself and allow for natural, daily variations. After my yoga, I work out on a cross-country skiing machine or a treadmill for a while, to raise my metabolism, burn some calories, and keep my heart in shape.

I leave the oil from my self-massage on my skin and in my hair while I exercise. This allows my skin, hair, and scalp to become wonderfully conditioned with oil, while the energizing aroma wakes up my body and helps my circulation. I feel greatly invigorated at this point.

SHOWER SCRUB

Now it's shower time. (Or, if I've been a good time manager, it could be bath time, and I can just relax into the water and some great aromatics and do my affirmations and meditation right in the bathtub.) Just think about how much we have already done in the morning before our shower! This is when I wash out the excess oil from my hair. That oil, by the way, is the best hair and scalp conditioner I have found. Putting deep-penetrating essential oils in a jojoba base on dry hair is the best way to lubricate the hair at every layer. Jojoba is the best oil for the hair since it most closely resembles the skin's own oil, sebum.

After I've washed my hair, I put a conditioner on it that seals in whatever moisture is left from the oil. I clean my body with an energizing wash. While in the shower, it's important not just to wash, but to exfoliate the skin, with an exfoliating scrub. I love how this feels, and it also stimulates and rejuvenates the skin.

JOJOBA HEAVEN

While my skin is still wet, I moisturize it with a combination of energizing and calming oils, preferably with a jojoba or a clarified jojoba base. Jojoba is the best choice of oil, but it's expensive. Some fine alternatives are sesame oil, grape seed oil, olive oil, hemp oil, borage oil, wheat germ oil, and sandalwood oil. Those who don't like aromas don't need to put fragrances in. Those who do like aromas should put in those essential oils that calm and that stimulate nurturing thoughts and feelings for them. I love plant fragrances, and I tend to mix in some very expensive ones, like rose and jasmine, because being in this business I have the luxury of doing so. Other favorites of mine that are much more reasonable are rosemary, bergamot, lavender, thyme, eucalyptus, lemon, orange, frankincense, chamomile sauvage, blue chamomile, and lavender green, from the leaves of the plant. I try to use stimulating and relaxing oils together, for a balance. Usually, and only when my skin is not dry, I dilute the mixture with some grain alcohol, to make it thinner and less viscous. After my body drinks up this fragrant mixture, which is also an antiseptic and deodorant, my skin feels like silk for the rest of the day, and my mind starts out from a calm, cleansed place.

REJUVENATING REFLECTIONS

It's time to face ourselves in the mirror. This is a time when men can do their shaving, and both men and women can do some facial treatments, such as toning and moisturizing. This is also a good moment to do additional facial acupressure, holding the pressure points until pulsations indicate that blood is flowing more aggressively through that area.

Caring for your complexion is not just important for women. Men need to cleanse, tone, exfoliate, and moisturize their skin, too. Regardless of gender, we all need to protect our faces from the sun, free radicals, and the weather; so each morning we should nourish them with products that are pleasing to our bodies and minds.

That said, I must confess that I do not always practice what I preach; I am not very good about tending to my face, in terms of toning, exfoliating, moisturizing, and wearing sunblock. I would probably have a lot fewer wrinkles if I were better about it. I do shade myself from the sun with a hat when I go out, and I try to avoid the sun from about 11 A.M. until 3 P.M., when the ultraviolet rays are strongest.

When I face the mirror in the morning, I do mirror-mind exercises, in which I program myself into a positive mode. Here I connect with my faith, in myself and my spiritual beliefs, and reinforce all of them. One exercise I do, which I learned from my teacher, Swami Rama, entails looking at myself in the mirror, and gazing with my right eye into my left eye while silently giving myself positive affirmations. This helps my creative side to influence my practical, analytical side. Next, I focus on the space between my eyebrows and visualize carrying out all the things I need to do in order to follow through on my affirmations, and then I visualize myself manifesting them. That little spot between my eyebrows becomes a mini–movie screen.

But this exercise is not the only approach to facing ourselves in the mirror in the morning. You can devise your own special practice for reflecting in the mirror on what it is you want from yourself each day, and visualizing yourself acting on your intentions.

Sometimes, after doing some mirroring exercises, I'll do my morning meditation right there in the bathroom.

MEDITATION-MINDED

In addition to in the mirror, I also practice my meditation in a special area I have created for myself. It is appointed with things I like to look at and aromas that stimulate nurturing feelings. You can create a special place just for your mirroring and meditation if you'd like, but it is by no means necessary. It ultimately matters a lot less where these two rituals take place than that they do take place, for sure, before we move on to the rest of our day.

HAIR, HAIR

While I'm still at the mirror, though, I often dry and style my hair. In the winter, I use a hair dryer, but when the weather is warmer, I just towel it dry. When it comes to my own hair styling, even though I was a hairdresser for many, many years, I am very low-maintenance. (When I'm on the road, I cut my own hair with the tiny scissors inside my Swiss Army knife!) For you, I recommend styling with products that are right for your particular type of hair and the desired texture.

At this point, women can put on an exfoliant, then a moisturizer followed by makeup, except for their lipstick, which goes on after breakfast. Men can put on a sun block foundation, with or without color, too. The makeup and sun block you use should be natural, with as few petrochemicals as possible, and without carcinogens. Petrochemicals put stress on the wearer and the environment; carcinogens are deadly.

BALANCED BREAKFAST BOOST

I tend to eat breakfast before getting dressed to leave the house, but these two practices can be reversed. I recommend a good, healthy breakfast, with a balance of protein, carbohydrate, fiber, and healthy essential fatty acids. For those who don't have time every day for a leisurely breakfast, there are nutritional powders that have the right balance of those things you need to keep your body healthy. Mixed with water, juice, or soy milk, or blended with whole fruits, these powders make drinks that are a delicious, filling way to get what I need into my system quickly. Of course, as often as possible, a slow, well-balanced meal with a soothing cup of organic herbal tea or green tea is preferable.

DRESSED AND READY

Now I get dressed for the day. All the things I've done up to this point have given me a feeling of optimism and well-being that affects my self-esteem positively. My ritual gives me the motivation and the creativity to look my best and go out in a good mood about myself, ready to face the day.

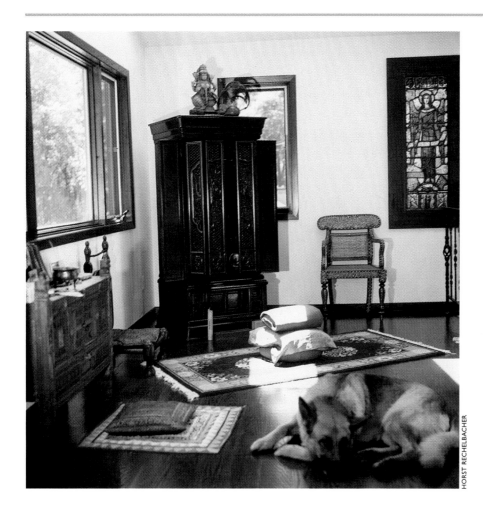

HORST RECHELBACHER

MY HAVEN

I have created a very elaborate meditation seat for myself, in a quiet spot on a balcony above my bedroom. I attribute the elaborateness to the fact that I was raised Catholic, a religion that includes lots of objects and imagery in its complex rituals.

I sit atop a variety of small pillows, each of which has meaning to me, that I have picked up in my travels around the world. On those pillows, I face a large altar that is an antique Buddhist meditation chest I found in China. It has lots of drawers, which I have filled with journals, incense and other sources of fragrance, candles, gifts I've received from religious leaders and shamans from many countries, Catholic worship objects such as rosary beads, and stones from a cave in the Himalayas where my teacher, Swami Rama, prayed. Displayed on the shelves are photographs of people who have left their bodies but still influence my life every day, including my teacher, my mother, and my father.

Because of sense memory response, all of these objects contribute to a feeling of bliss that makes meditation easy in this special little haven.

YOUR HAVEN

Create a special place for yourself where you can calmly, quietly meditate. Add any or all of the following items:

- candles
- incense
- a mirror
- a photo of a person, place, or thing that has spiritual meaning for you personally
- a rug
- a pillow

DRIVING DELIGHT

Those of us who drive to work can make the transition from home to the office a much more pleasant one by using aromatherapy in the car. I do. There are diffusers designed specifically for cars. Breathing in scents that arouse nurturing feelings is a nice way to prepare to work and to keep any driving stress to a minimum.

Midday

AROMA ENERGIZER

In the middle of the morning, when it's not quite lunchtime and I am often beginning to lag or to feel anxious because of some anticipated meeting at work, a nice ritual is breathing in some energizing or calming aromas. I frequently diffuse oils or incense in diffusers, just sniff a bottle of oil, drop some oil into some old potpourri, or dab some oil onto a handkerchief and sniff it as I need to.

LET-GO LUNCH

I find taking a real lunch break very important. I try not to eat while I work, because to me, eating is a sacred experience that must be noticed and enjoyed. I won't ever eat at my desk, because if I did there would be no boundary between my private life and my work. I get out of the office to eat, go to the cafeteria or to a park even if it's only for twenty minutes, and experience my food. I make a point of having a well-balanced lunch, with a nice selection of protein, fiber, and essential fatty acids.

INVIGORATING INVENTORY

If there's time left after I'm done eating, I take a walk and do my midday inventory and affirmations. If I can't do that at lunch time, I take a break a little later in the day for it. At this time, I reflect on what's taken place already, and how what has transpired brings me closer to fulfilling my goals for the day, and my larger goals, too. I use this time to evaluate how to go forward with the rest of the day.

HIGH-NOON HYGIENE

Flossing, brushing my teeth, and scraping my tongue after lunch will improve the condition of my gums and teeth, and remove toxins from my mouth that can slow me down. Yet even though I know this—and even though I *do* carry around floss and a toothbrush—I am still not con-

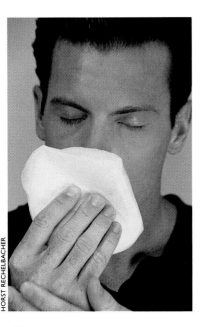

*T*ry an aroma energizer—just a few drops of your favorite oil on a hand-kerchief.

sistent about oral hygiene after lunch. I know I need to improve in this area.

EXERCISE ESCAPE

Some days, I use my lunch break, or part of it, for exercise. Companies that have on-site gymnasiums, like AVEDA does, make it easy for people to enjoy midday workouts. I also like to take invigorating walks at lunch, be it at home or at work, here or abroad.

POSTLUNCH PICK-ME-UP

In the latter part of the afternoon, I often need to revive my energy and my spirit by doing some self-massage, some yoga or tai chi, some breathing exercises, or a combination of all three. Even just five or ten minutes of any of these will increase circulation and help the body cleanse itself of the toxins that come from and cause the day's stress. If I take a short break to work these practices in, they give me the energy I need to get through the rest of the workday in a less stressful way.

SMELL SENSATION

Sniffing an energizing or stimulating aroma is another very easy way I have found to revive energy late in the workday.

A MOMENT'S MIST

I also like to spritz my face with a rose-water-based skin toner as an afternoon boost. This is not only lovely to smell and refreshing to the mind, it is also great for rejuvenating and moisturizing my skin.

TRANQUIL TRANSITION

I fill my ride home with aromatherapy, just as I did on the ride to work. Breathing in fragrances I love is a nice way to ease the transition from work back to home.

Evening

BEAUTIFUL BOUNDARIES

I like to clarify the boundary between work and home by changing into clothes that are comfortable but attractive to me and to my partner. We need to remember that we want to be beautiful for ourselves and those close to us—not just for the people we work with or see at the market.

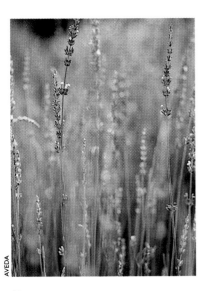

*L*avender oil added to an evening bath makes it even more relaxing.

DINER'S DELIGHT

I look toward dinnertime as a time of sharing food and conversation. Again, we want to have a meal with a good balance of carbohydrate, protein, fiber, and essential fatty acids. And we want to eat in a relaxed fashion. No standing at the counter and picking at things. I find it rejuvenating to sit and be mindful of what I'm eating, and of who is present with me. It is acknowledging and cherishing these moments that give our lives meaning and depth.

EVENING EXERCISE

After I eat in the evening I try to do some exercise, but preferably nothing too invigorating. For the evening I like activities like yoga, walking, or going for a leisurely bike ride. Many people work out in the evening, because they really have no other time. But because we're soon going to be getting ready for bed, our exercise at this time of the day shouldn't stimulate us too much.

MEDITATION MOMENT

Now I move on to meditate and release my goals. Retreat to the special spiritual areas you have created for yourself, even if only for five minutes, to meditate and just be.

EVENSONG EVALUATION

It's inventory time again. Now, after meditation, I reflect on the day I've just completed, evaluate what worked and what didn't, what aroused feelings of pain and what aroused feelings of being nurtured, and plan tomorrow. I have found that writing these things in a journal is helpful toward turning my thoughts into actions.

RELAXING RINSE

If there is enough time, I find a bath is a very relaxing ritual to add to any day. That bath can be an experience of aromatherapy, with essential oils placed in the water to bring about a positive, relaxed state of mind. It's also a wonderful alternative place to do your mirroring and meditation, since the warm water and natural aromas calm the body and still the mind.

CALM CLEANSING

Cleansing the face of the day's makeup and grime is key for men and women (note that many men are wearing foundation with sunblock these days). Before bed, I use a calming facial wash. Then I apply an exfoliant and massage a moisturizer into my face—when I'm being good. Just because I don't always follow these last steps doesn't mean you shouldn't. Exfoliate and moisturize, and I promise you'll have fewer wrinkles than I do!

TEETH TIME

It's time to brush, floss, and scrape again.

PAMPERING PARTNERS

Now comes the fun part. My partner and I give each other massages, with jojoba and essential oils, or a ready-made calming massage oil that both she and I like. This is not only enjoyable, it is absolutely necessary. Everyone should learn the way to massage properly and should massage their partners for at least fifteen minutes a night. Aside from the physiological benefits, partner massaging strengthens relationships. It is about nurturing and spoiling your partner; it is an interactive act of love and caring. The intent of love can be transferred through all our senses, and touch is one of them. Partner massage need not be limited to romantic partners. It can be done between parent and child, or other family members. What a lovely way to interact with a parent, or someone who is elderly and needs help with skin care, or even a neighbor who is lonely and needs to be nurtured.

BACK TO BED

Time for bed. And I look forward to doing it all again the next day.

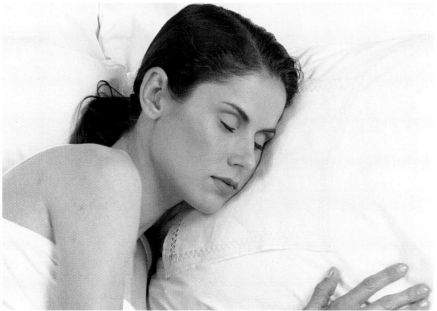

HORST RECHELBACHER

Calming oils diffused in your bedroom ease you to sleep. Place a hankerchief dabbed with your favorite soothing scent on your pillow.

THE 24-HOUR DAILY TIME WHEEL

Are there ever enough hours in a day? Here's a time wheel to help you understand how some of the new habits I've suggested can fit into your busy schedule. You can manage your time differently, of course. But I find that wheels like this can be useful in doing daily planning, to understand where all your time is going.

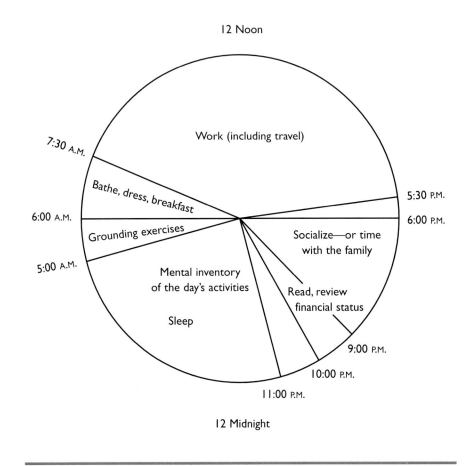

12 Noon

7:30 A.M.

Work (including travel)

5:30 P.M.

Bathe, dress, breakfast

6:00 A.M.

6:00 P.M.

Grounding exercises

Socialize—or time
with the family

5:00 A.M.

Mental inventory
of the day's activities

Read, review
financial status

Sleep

9:00 P.M.

10:00 P.M.

11:00 P.M.

12 Midnight

YOUR TURN

Whatever set of habits you decide to design for yourself, make sure that the components you choose feel right to you and are truly nurturing to your body, mind, and spirit. One of the most important things about your rituals is that you enjoy them. You want to enjoy these nurturing habits, and look forward to them, so that you will be inclined to keep them in your life, even on the days when you are feeling lazy or reluctant. Our rituals can and should be modified until they fit us just right, for this very reason. This set of activities you bring together is no good to anyone if you don't practice it. So, make it something you love.

It's important that we like our nurturing daily habits because it's also important that we practice them regularly. They need really to become habits, things that get to be second nature to us. We already have so many habits of which we're not aware, and many of which cause us stress. Now, we need to replace them with positive practices of which we're conscious. In the same time that it takes us to carry out our less healthy, unconscious routines, we can carry out our healthy, conscious ones.

As we get used to these new habits, we should increasingly surround our-selves with the activities, items, and people we have chosen, the things that nurture us through sensory perception. We must surround ourselves with that which inspires healthy thoughts within us. We need to practice healthy thinking on a daily, even a momentary basis. And if a thought that doesn't nurture enters the mind, offer it to whatever divine gods you worship, who-ever they are, and trust them.

The challenge is to be conscious at every moment and to have faith in this process. The rejuvenation sciences are real, and they should be taken very seriously. Know that these are principles by which some great people on this planet have lived. They are nonviolent principles, nonviolent to ourselves and the world with which we have a relationship as well. When we switch from stressful to nurturing habits, we are practicing nonviolence. We are nurturing—making friends with any negative feelings we might be carrying within us. In doing so, we diffuse that negative energy and open ourselves once more to the world.

The object of the game is to reduce, release, and eliminate as much stress as possible, and to restore harmony with nurturing. What nurtures strength-ens. A self-nurtured state strengthens immunity. What stresses weakens.

We need to heal ourselves continually from stress. There are new stresses, physical, emotional, and spiritual, every day. And there is no limit to the benefits we can receive from crafting and adhering to a set of de-stressing, nurturing daily rituals that's just right for each of us. I've shared mine with you; now it's time for you to build your own.

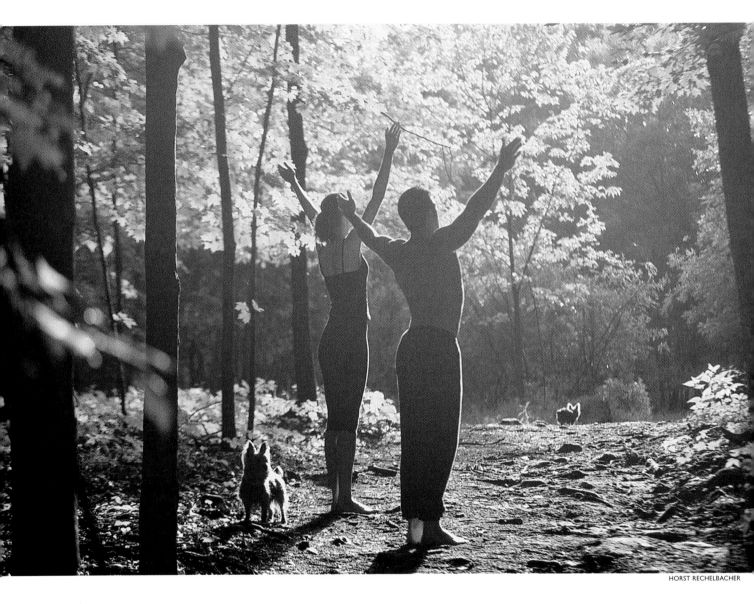

HORST RECHELBACHER

Oh What a Beautiful Morning

Welcoming Every New Day

The early morning hath gold in its mouth.

—Benjamin Franklin

HOW MANY OF US ACTUALLY LOOK FORWARD TO GETTING up and out of bed in the morning? It is common for many people to cling to sleep and inactivity, and then approach the day with reluctance. This is one habit.

An alternate and more positive habit we can adopt is recognizing each day as a gift and a new set of opportunities. Each morning that we awake, rejuvenate, tune into our senses, and prepare to meet the world is another chance for growth, fulfillment, and passage into the zone of bliss.

Changing habits can be easier and more pleasurable than it might seem at first. When each of us realizes that all the positive practices we undertake have a nurturing, harmonizing, and restorative effect on our whole being, it becomes less difficult to get onto this new path. As we experience the enjoyment and discovery that grows with the practice of each new habit, it becomes less difficult to stick to a plan of action. To tune into all the benefits of positive changes we make in our lives, it helps to practice mindfulness, paying close, pointed attention to what we think and feel in each moment, being fully aware of all our senses and our breath.

So, here we are, at the beginning of a new day. We're ready to explore and develop our relationships with the things and people around us, our senses, and ourselves. Each one of us can do this, in our own way. Let's take a closer look at the recommended nurturing practices for the morning, in the order I first presented them in Chapter 5. What are the different options we can choose from within each of the practices? What are their benefits? How do they affect our senses? All of these questions help us to see the physical, mental, and spiritual advantages of incorporating these new habits into our days. In the chapters ahead, I'll address the practices recommended for midday, evening, and special occasions as well. In the end, you will have a wealth of nurturing options for your mind and your body to tailor to any time or situation you may face. Look at this chapter and the ones that follow as a grand menu, a smorgasbord of practices from which you can design the routine that works best for you. Feel free to redesign it as often as you like.

RISE AND SHINE

Before we can greet the day with gusto and enthusiasm we need to adopt an attitude of faith in the universe and whatever we choose to believe in. We must have an appreciation for each day. In other words, we need consciously to decide to wake up on the *right* side of the bed, and take steps to do so.

Part of that, for me, is making a mental space for myself to reflect on my life and to feel gratitude at the moment I wake up. Before I get out of my bed, I like to think positively about why I am here in this life, and what is good about it. I want my first thought of the day to be a positive one. This can set an optimistic tone for the whole day.

Bear in mind, if you are going to add new practices to your day, you will likely need to start getting up earlier than you are accustomed to. This doesn't have to be a source of grumpiness. Think of getting up earlier as creating special time for yourself, time to treat yourself better and to nurture yourself. Even if we just awaken a half hour earlier than usual, we can have time for several beneficial practices, such as meditation, self-massage, and personal inventory. That time is not a sacrifice but a gift to ourselves.

OPEN WIDE

Morning breath is nature's way of telling us that we've got to get the toxins out of our mouths, and fast. Overnight, while we sleep, our mouths accumulate all sorts of bacteria, friendly and unfriendly, along with lots of toxins.

Although a certain brand of mouthwash presents its product, in commercials, as the ultimate antidote to morning breath and germs, it is important to realize that rinsing alone isn't nearly enough to do the trick. Sure, rinsing with a minty mouthwash will improve our breath. But that's merely a cosmetic move. Rinsing doesn't effectively deal with the germs below the gum line, between teeth, and in the tiny crevices of our tongues.

It's a good idea to rinse with a natural mouthwash that is either made up of or includes in its ingredients tea tree, peppermint, lemon, or Roman chamomile oil, essential oils that are very good for teeth and gums, and that have natural antibacterial properties. There are also some toothpastes on the market that contain these oils. These can usually be found in health food stores and food co-ops. If you're going to formulate your own mouthwash or toothpaste, remember that too much of these oils can be toxic. Be sure you know how much to use.

Flossing is a good idea, too. While flossing is much more necessary later in the day, to remove any food that gets stuck between our teeth, it helps to floss more than once a day. The benefit: stronger, healthier gums and jaw bones.

Don't forget your tongue in your hygiene routine for your mouth. Most people take care of their teeth and gums in the morning, but not everyone

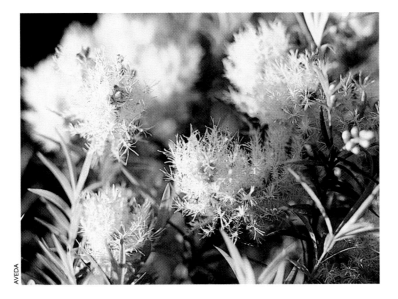

AVEDA

Cleanse your body with deep breaths. Cleanse your breath with tea tree. Its antiseptic and antifungal properties will help keep your breath fresh all day.

Fresh breath comes tongue first!

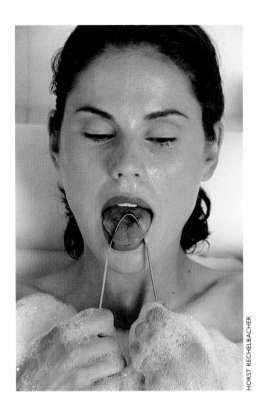

HORST RECHELBACHER

pays attention to the tongue. We use our tongues for so much—for tasting, for talking, even kissing—yet it doesn't occur to many of us to make sure they're clean and free of harmful germs.

The tongue is a virtual sponge, receiving and holding on to bacteria and toxins. Overnight, when our mouths are closed for hours, is when many of these little visitors accumulate. That's why it's important to clean our tongues with either a tongue scraper or just a spoon. The need to clean our tongues is receiving greater awareness, so tongue scrapers are becoming more available at health food stores, small apothecaries, and even national drug chains. Scraping the tongue adds maybe another thirty to forty-five seconds to our morning regimen and keeps our mouths fresher and cleaner throughout the day. Why not do it?

THE FIRST BREATHS

Before we begin our next practice, morning self-massage, let's do some breathing exercises. After a night of sleeping and drifting apart, these simple, focused breaths link our mind and body firmly together. Since breath is the connector between body and mind, we need to tune into it before we can really approach other nurturing and healing practices most effectively. While breath comes naturally to our bodies, it can also be altered and controlled with thought and concentration. This awareness of our breath can be a key factor in making life changes and in all sorts of healing. Relaxed, effective breathing can help us ward off many kinds of diseases by helping us decrease stress and ease its demands on our immune systems.

Some of the breathing exercises I recommend for this time of day are simple: controlled, slow breathing and alternate nostril breathing.

For controlled, slow breathing:

- Sit comfortably on a chair or on the floor. Sit upright with a very straight back.
- Begin with a deep, slow breath, drawing in as much air as you can to fill completely your body cavity from the bottom up.
- Let your mind imagine where this breath travels to in your body. Once you have filled your body with air, hold it and be aware of it.
- Then, slowly, with the intention of emptying the air out from the bottom of your stomach on up, release the breath, exhaling little by little until you are empty of air once again. Do this at least ten times.

When you're done with that exercise, you might move on to alternate nostril breathing, one of the best exercises for integrating mind and body, as well as balancing left brain and right brain, and yin and yang. Alternate nostril breathing is a great way to release anger, as well.

For alternate nostril breathing:

- Using the thumb and ring finger of one hand, first close off one nostril as you breath slowly into the other nostril.
- Then switch fingers to close off the other nostril, and exhale through the opposite one.
- Inhale through the open nostril, and then close it off before exhaling through the other. Do this at least three times on each side.

After you've completed both breathing exercises, take note of how you feel. I think you'll notice that you're more awake, calm, and relaxed than you usually are at this time of the morning—or any time for that matter. It is important to reflect on how you feel at this moment because the positive sensation is what will help you get out of bed and embrace the day in the same fashion tomorrow. Once we've connected with our breath, we're ready to connect with the rest of our body, or to do mirroring and meditation. Actually, we're ready for anything!

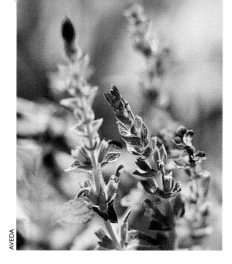

AVEDA

Healing Touch

Techniques for Self-Massage

It is shameful for a man to rest in ignorance of the structure of his own body, especially when the knowledge of it mainly conduces to his welfare, and directs his application of his own powers.

—Philip Schwarzert

TO SOME PEOPLE, SELF-MASSAGE MIGHT SEEM LIKE MORE of a frivolous indulgence than a necessary daily practice. But massage doesn't just feel good. It does us a great deal of deeper good. Recent studies reveal how necessary this hands-on practice is to achieving optimal health and immunity. For instance, we now know that massaging the chest area near the sternum encourages the maturation of T cells, which promotes the production of neuropeptides, immune system building blocks. This is just one of the benefits massage has been found to have.

When we practice self-massage, we

- improve our circulation
- raise our energy level
- increase our immunity
- ease the emission of toxins from our muscles and lymph nodes
- moisten our skin
- balance the five elements within us
- heighten our awareness of our bodies, our sense of touch, and our relationship with ourselves

That's a lot to accomplish in five or ten minutes of careful kneading and manipulating. In fact, daily self-massage is one of the most important habits we can adopt. It can be practiced just once a day or several times a day. For example, while at work, we can stimulate our energy and clear our minds with just a little bit of self-massage on the scalp and body. Before we go to bed, we can work our bodies again—or we can stimulate our many physical systems and add to feelings of intimate nurturing by having our partners or family members do it for us.

In the morning, I like to use a massage oil that has energizing properties to help me start my day. Some examples of oils that are energizing are peppermint, eucalyptus, and ylang-ylang. I like to use jojoba or evening primrose oil as a base, but they are very expensive and pure sesame, olive, grape seed, hemp, or coconut are very good oils for massage as well.

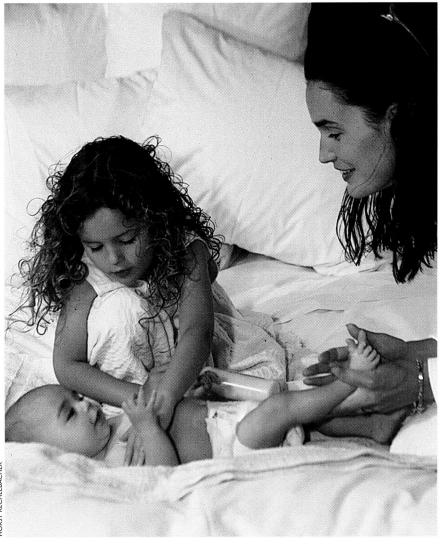

Massage, a nurturing, bonding, healing pleasure

Jojoba provides the perfect oil for massage. Bearing a remarkable similarity to the oil produced by our own glands, it is well absorbed by and extremely beneficial to our skin.

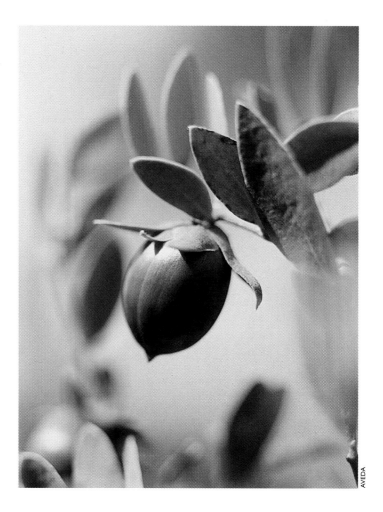

AVEDA

In the chapter on aromatherapy, I will discuss the nature of essential oils, where they come from, and how to choose the fragrances that are best for you. In the chapter on healing, I'll make clear which oils work best in treating certain ailments. Be sure to read both of these sections before choosing the oils you use for massage.

To begin the morning self-massage, we put our pure oil combined with our essential oils of choice into our hair, in preparation for a face and scalp massage. Especially if you have long hair, brush the oil through to the ends and twist your hair up and secure it with a barrette or a tie of some sort. It might seem unusual to be putting oil into your hair as I suggest, but it is really good for your hair and scalp in general, and is an important component to the body massage that comes next. Don't rush to wash the oil out. Leave it in. The very best way to condition your hair is to put oil in it before it is wet. Trust me on this; after all, I got my start in the health and beauty business as a hairstylist. Once your hair is moist with oil, you're ready for your scalp and face massage. Enjoy!

HEAD AND SHOULDERS

Here's how to do a self-facial and scalp massage:

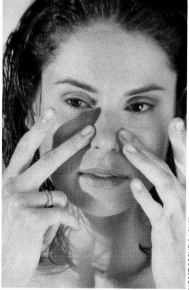

*E*ase your breath with a touch.

▸ Sit in a quiet place. Adjust yourself so you are sitting comfortably in your chair or on the floor. Relax your breathing.

▸ Rub hands together briskly until they feel warm.

▸ Apply both hands to cheeks and breathe deeply three times.

▸ Rub cheeks up and down until warm.

▸ Close your eyes, cover them with your palms, and hold this position. Breathe in and out several times. This will energize the regions around your eyes and relieve stress and tension there.

▸ Keeping eyes closed, use your index, middle, and ring fingers to press firmly on the bony ridge of the upper eye socket. Move from the inside of the ridge to the outside, away from your nose and toward your hairline. Then press the bones underneath the eyes. Repeat several times.

▸ If you are a contact lens wearer, skip this step, or only do it when you are not wearing your lenses. With eyes still closed, use the tips of your fingers and gently press the front of the eyeballs and quickly pull the fingers off. Repeat ten times. This will release tension from the eyes.

▸ Using the thumb and the index finger, pinch the bridge of the nose. Press deeply for ten seconds. Then detach by pulling your fingers away from your face. Repeat three to five times. This is a good remedy for relieving strain and fatigue in the eyes.

▸ Rub the sides of your nose up and down until they're warm. This will help to make your breathing smooth and steady.

▸ Massage the thin area between your nose and mouth with all four fingers of both hands. Use a circular motion, beginning in the center and working toward your cheeks. Repeat seven to ten times.

▸ Place your thumbs under your cheekbones, about a finger's width away from the sides of your nose. Rub in a circular motion for a moment. This will relieve any tension in your face that might be caused by sinus congestion.

▸ Press deeply under the lower jaw with the thumbs as if making deep indentations from underneath the ears to below the chin. Repeat three to five times. This movement will tone the skin and the muscles of the jaw.

▸ Use your index, middle, and ring fingers to press around your ears several times. This will increase circulation in the ear and improve your sense of balance.

▸ Using the thumbs and the index fingers, hold the tops of your ears, pulling upward. Then pull from the sides of your ears outward, and from the

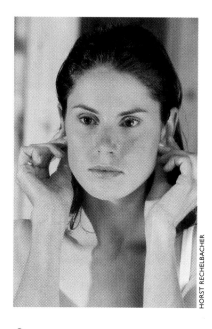

*S*timulate your chi with a gentle pull.

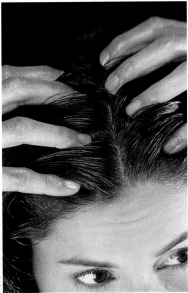

*E*ssential oils condition scalp and soul.

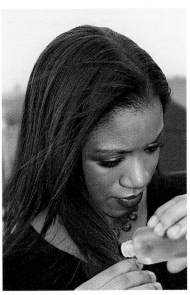

lobes downward. Repeat twice in each direction. This stimulates the flow of energy and assists in the elimination of toxins.

   » Place your hands, palms facing forward, behind the ears. Briskly strike the ears back and forth. Repeat ten to twenty times to increase blood circulation in the ears.

   » Knead your ears to fully awaken them, beginning at the earlobes, moving around the edge to the top of the ears, and then to the inner ears.

   » Cover your left ear with the right hand. With the first three fingers of your left hand, tap briskly on the back of your right hand, creating the sensation of sharp vibrations toward the inner ear. Tap in pairs and repeat ten pairs of taps on each ear. This exercise helps to stimulate the eardrum.

   » Using the index and middle finger, massage the temples. Rub in a circular motion for a minute or two. This will release tension and stagnated mental energy.

   » If you haven't already applied an oil composition to your scalp, do so now. This composition, a base oil with essential oils that are energizing, relaxing, or both, can be warmed in a dropper bottle in a sink of hot water at home. Using all fingers, vigorously massage the entire scalp with a strong, rapid back-and-forth "shampooing" motion. Continue for about one minute.

   » Next, briskly press the tips of all ten fingers into the scalp to stimulate circulation; repeat this motion moving from the front of the head, to the crown, to the back of the head, and then forward.

   » Perform therapeutic brushing working in all directions to stimulate the scalp and distribute the oil.

   » Perform pressure-point massage—working from the hairline to the crown in pie-shaped sections. Press the scalp between your thumbs to increase blood flow to the scalp.

   » Gently pull the hair at the roots. Brush out hair.

   » Tilt head to the left. With a loose fist, gently strike the right side of the neck. Repeat on the left side using right hand.

   » Tilt head forward and gently strike on the back of neck. Relax head fully forward then back several times. Repeat from side to side.

   » Rotate neck counterclockwise, three to five times, then clockwise three to five times.

   » Raise your shoulders, contracting them as much as possible, then releasing them quickly. Repeat this five times, releasing tension in your neck and shoulders and activating smooth functioning of your intestines.

   » Tilting your head to one side, press down and massage the opposite shoulder. Repeat on your other shoulder. This step will loosen tension and stiffness in your shoulders and back.

◗ Make a loose fist with one hand and pound the opposite shoulder (while head is still tilted away from the shoulder being pounded). Repeat ten to twenty times on each shoulder, then continue to pound the back of the neck at the top of the spine.

◗ Apply your palms to opposite shoulders and breathe in and out three times to harmonize the flow of energy throughout the body.

◗ Sit comfortably, resting your hands on your thighs. Close your eyes and let your mind and body relax. Breathe normally for a minute. Allow the

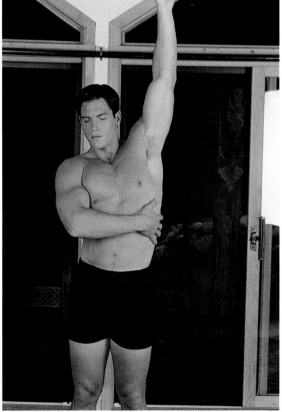

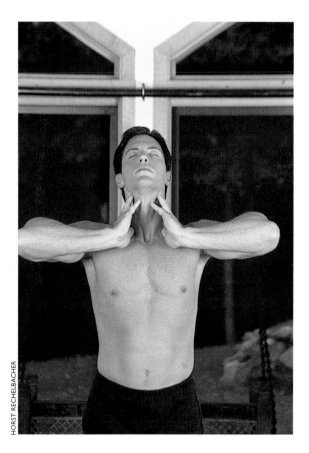

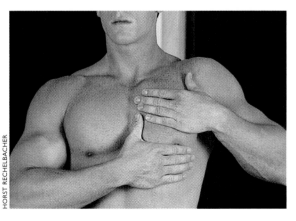

Smooth away kinks and night stiffness with effleurage, a gliding up-and-down motion on your arms, sides, and neck. Use petrissage, a circular motion, for massaging your chest, stomach, and joints.

energy to flow freely to every part of your body—to every tiny cell. See yourself radiating health and filled with a sense of well-being. Hold that image. Slowly open your eyes.

FROM THE NECK DOWN

For much of the rest of the body, from the shoulders down, there are two alternating motions used in self-massage: effleurage, a gliding up-and-down stroking motion; and petrissage, a circular motion.

‣ Rub your body from the shoulders down, by using effleurage, an up-and-down motion, on parts of limbs, and petrissage, circular motions, on joints. Linger for about a half minute on each part.

ABDOMEN

‣ Massage the abdomen in a circular motion, but be sure always to massage your stomach in a clockwise direction. That is the direction in which the fluids of digestion flow, and it is always best to work with the flow of things, rather than against it. This massage technique also assists lymphatic drainage.

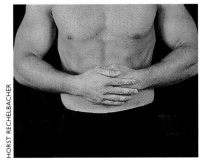

*G*et your juices flowing in the right direction: clockwise!

HANDS

Massage your hands in the following way:

‣ Begin by shaking your hands to get your circulation moving.
‣ Press the thumb of one hand into the palm of the other. Move your thumb along the palm, starting at the heel and sliding up between the fingers.
‣ Massage each palm in deep, circular motions, working from the heel of the hand toward the fingers.
‣ Squeeze the thumb, beginning at the base, pumping and squeezing to the end. Apply pressure to the base of the nail, to the tip, then squeeze the sides. Complete by pinching the tip.
‣ Find the pressure point between the thumb and the index finger by looking at the top of your hand, holding your hand flat and thumb in. You

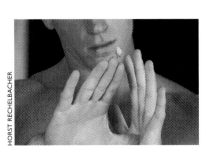

*G*ive yourself a hand massage.

will see a bump where your thumb meets the rest of your hand. Spread fingers and apply pressure to that point.

◗ Work through each finger from base to tip the same way you worked the thumb.

◗ Repeat massage on your other hand.

FEET

Each morning, when you do your self-massage, it's important to make sure you include your feet. If you're short on time, you can skimp on other areas, but try not to take shortcuts when it comes to the soles of your feet. Because of the reflexology relationship between your feet and all the other organs and glands of your body, your soles have a significance, and massaging them has an increased effect.

You don't necessarily need to perform a whole reflexology massage each day. That can be done less frequently, once a week or so. Here's a simpler routine that's good for every day:

◗ Massage a replenishing body moisturizer into the foot. You can use a lotion, or simply a base oil with some essential oils mixed in.

◗ Stretch your foot one direction at a time, stretching in all directions.

◗ Using your knuckles, massage the entire sole of your foot.

◗ Massage the arch of your foot using an effleurage motion—gliding strokes—working from the heel to the big toe.

◗ Separate the big toe and the second toe. Using your index finger, massage between the toes, making large, circular motions.

◗ Using the same motion, massage from the heel to the second toe, and massage in circular motions at the base of the toe. Repeat, working from the heel to the third, fourth, and fifth toes.

◗ Massage between the ligaments and tendons on the top of your foot with your fingers working from the toes up toward the ankle.

◗ Squeeze the big toe, starting at the base. Pump and squeeze toward the tip. Apply pressure at the base of the nail, then at the tip of the sides. Complete by pinching off the tip. Finish each of your toes on this foot with this sequence.

◗ Repeat massage on your other foot.

Of course, we also nurture our minds through our sense of smell when we administer a self-massage. When we do any kind of massage using an

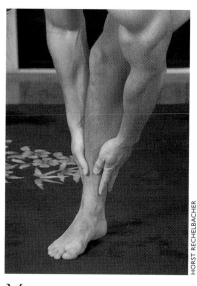

*M*assage from knee to ankle with effleurage, a long flowing massage stroke.

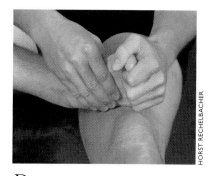

*D*eep foot massage has full-body effects.

Eucalyptus invigorates any massage. In addition, it clears congestion and is good for colds, coughs, and other respiratory disorders.

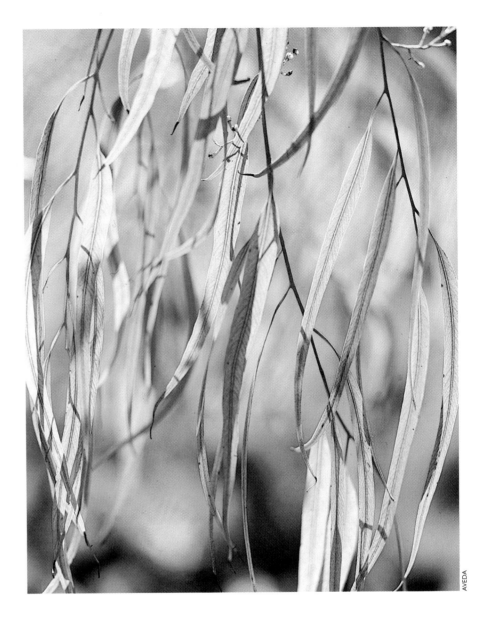

AVEDA

essential oil or combination of oils, including those with fragrances that arouse nurturing feelings in us, we also experience the benefits of aromatherapy. So we are soothing our minds through our noses as we also soothe and work our flesh with our fingers. There's yet another mind-body connection, which awaits us in the section ahead.

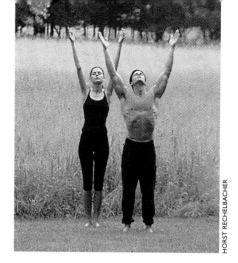

HORST RECHELBACHER

Graceful Motion

Yoga is for everyone, for the West as well as the East. One would not say the telephone is not for the East because it was invented in the West. Through yoga, we can build a direct line to God.

— YOGANANDA

WHEN WE WERE CHILDREN, WE DIDN'T MIND EXERCISING. Most of us probably didn't even think of exercise as exercise. We thought of riding our bicycles and running around as *playing*, and, as a result, it had a buoyant effect on our spirits. It's a good idea to reconnect with that playful spirit from childhood before we approach new habits regarding movement, especially those of us who usually approach it with dread. It's also inspiring to contemplate the many benefits that come from a regular regimen of body movements, including stretching, low-impact exercise, and aerobic exercise. We increase our heart rate and our immunity, raise our metabolism, manage our weight, lower our blood pressure, release stress and toxins, tone our muscles, strengthen the connection among mind, body, and spirit, prolong our youthfulness, build good cholesterol, and generally lengthen our lives. If those incentives don't inspire you, just think about the healthy glow that results from a half hour of yoga, followed by a brisk two-mile walk.

Like so many of the choices we make regarding our sets of daily rituals, choosing the sort of exercise that's right for each of us is very personal. We must each select activities that make us feel good and with which we're comfortable.

Making this choice is often easier when we confer with a coach or mentor. This person can be a yoga teacher or personal trainer, and can come from a health club, yoga studio, or private practice. These people certainly don't need to be with us every day, but they can help us design exercise programs that are right for us, individually. They can help get us started on the right track, one to which we are most likely to stay committed.

It is also a good idea to take into consideration our elemental makeups, or Ayurvedic doshas, when designing an exercise regimen. People who have high air and space constitutions, or vata, will be more inclined to do highly aerobic activities, like running, but should instead do lower-impact, calmer exercises. Conversely, those with high earth and water constitutions, or kapha, will be inclined to be slow and sedentary, but should instead balance out their nature with high-energy aerobic activity. People with high fire constitutions, or pitta, will be best off with a moderate level of aerobic exercise.

One exercise that is recommended for everyone is brisk walking. In fact, doctors recommend that people of all elemental makeups take two brisk walks a day, although those walks can be interchanged with other modes of exercise.

In addition, we can all benefit from a combination of different types of movement at different times of the day. Before we engage in aerobic activity, which is best done in the morning or afternoon, it is good to first awaken and connect our minds and bodies with yoga or tai chi stretches and postures. Then, after our aerobic exercise, I suggest cooling down again with a more passive exercise. What I try to do each morning, after my *pranayama*, or breathing exercises, and my self-massage, is some sit-ups and push-ups. I like these exercises because with them I use my own weight for lifting. Then I'll walk briskly and use some cardiovascular machines, such as a treadmill or a cross-country skiing machine followed by a cooling-down sequence. I follow the cool down with some slow breathing exercises that help me make the transition into a contemplative state, for meditation and mirroring.

In the afternoon, we can do some yoga or tai chi again, even at work, to reconnect the mind and body, and to invigorate ourselves without getting all worked up and sweaty. In the evening, after dinner, a gentle stroll, a bike ride, or some stretching is a good way to keep the blood flowing without reenergizing the body too close to bedtime.

OUR PURPOSE

While playing competitive sports can be a part of our daily movement ritual, it is important that, above all, the purpose of our exercise is not to conquer others. We can win at a game of tennis, even without making it our goal to beat the other person, by changing our focus and playing the game with the aim of improving our strength and energy, and working our bodies. We even can win that game *and* help our opponent to improve, instead of lording a victory of points over him or her.

We should never engage in exercise for the sake of competing with others, whether it's people in our exercise class or our partners. Daily movement should not be about who can prove he or she is stronger or more beautiful. Motion is a component in strengthening our relationship with the self and, through that, our relationships with others. We truly benefit from it when we are focused on our own growth, and when we are willing to help others work toward their growth. That holds true for every aspect of a healthy society.

THE PERFECT UNION

Of all forms of movement, yoga is one of the most universally recommended, and one of the most effective, from a holistic standpoint. The word *yoga* refers not only to a certain type of body movement; it is defined as the union of mind, body, and spirit. That connection is the purpose of the tradition of movement known as yoga. Studying and practicing yoga heals and bonds all three sectors of our being. It requires the effort of all three, and it balances and unites them in the process.

There are many different types of yoga movement that are taught in yoga studios all over the world. Some, like Japa meditation yoga, are more mind-oriented. Karma yoga is the yoga of emotion, which deals with past healing through emotion and through meditating on the well-being of others. For our purposes in this book, though, I will mostly refer to positions from what is known as Hatha yoga, a type of yoga that leans toward physical exercise, stretching, and breathing.

Yoga is generally a slow-moving form of exercise. When we practice yoga, we are taught to be slow about entering, holding, and releasing ourselves from each posture. There are poses designed to work every muscle and joint in the body, and to stimulate the body's cardiovascular, digestive, nervous, and endocrine systems. Among the goals of yoga are the symmetrical balancing and aligning of the musculoskeletal system, and promoting optimal body function so that we are physically and emotionally free of stress.

Even those who have been practicing yoga for many years find some stretches and postures difficult to achieve and hold. Growth occurs in yoga when we feel pain, use the pain as a teacher, and move past it to the next level of difficulty. The same is true in every other area of our lives, and that reflects the universality of the lessons of yoga.

It is important to make sure that we listen to our bodies as we do our yoga. While we need to work through discomfort in order to develop our skill, we must be careful not to strain ourselves too much at once. It's a delicate balance. Yoga practice can be modified to suit anyone's level of ability, regardless of age or physical fitness. Before designing your own daily yoga rituals for home practice, it's a good idea to take a beginner yoga class, or maybe even a private yoga session, to acquaint yourself with some of the basic postures and how they're supposed to look and feel.

It is also important to learn to breathe properly during yoga practice. You must breathe through your nose, rather than your mouth. Your nose and sinus tissue act as important filters, removing impurities from the air, and conditioning the temperature of the air as it enters your body.

In addition, it should be noted that coordinating breath and movement is key to reaping the benefits of yoga or of any mode of exercise. Movements should be executed on the exhalation of a breath, rather than on the inhalation. And the breath should never be held while you are moving.

YOGA PRACTICE

Not everyone has the time to do a half hour or more of yoga each day, and although such a commitment does produce wonderful results, this is not necessary. You can receive benefits from practicing just a few postures each day, one or more times a day. You can do a longer session in the morning, and then just a few postures at work to free the mind and boost energy. What I want to impress upon you is that any amount of yoga you do will help. If possible, do just a bit rather than none at all because you feel what you can fit in your schedule is too little. It's simply not. Do what you can. Before beginning practice, heed the following cautions and tips:

1. If you are under the care of a doctor or chiropractor, discuss your intention to practice yoga with her or him.

2. Empty your bladder and bowels before practicing. (The postures will lead to regularity of the bowels.)

3. Practice your yoga in a clean, quiet spot, at a time of the day during which you can be relaxed and concentrate on your movements.

4. Wait at least two hours after a heavy meal before practicing.

5. Wear comfortable clothing that will allow free movement. Shorts and a T-shirt or footless leotards work well. Cotton is a preferable fiber, as it allows the body to breathe. Always practice barefoot.

6. Breathe gently and quietly through your nose during your practice. Smooth breathing is more important than deep breathing. Make all of your movements on the exhalation rather than the inhalation, and never hold your breath.

7. Keep your eyes and mind quietly attentive to check alignment and make adjustments.

8. Never bounce your way into a stretch! Attempting to lengthen a muscle by bouncing or jerking activates the dynamic stretch reflex, which is the mechanism built into the muscle spindles to prevent overstretching and injury. Bouncing actually tightens the muscle and counteracts the desired effect of stretching.

9. Eliminate extra effort. Work only the muscles necessary to hold the pose; notice and relax any tension in the eyes, face, tongue, jaw, neck, throat, shoulders, and abdomen.

10. If you feel a sharp or fierce pain in any pose, slowly leave the pose. Examine and adjust the pose to lessen the stretch, and check your alignment. If the pain persists, seek advice from an experienced yoga teacher.

11. Be persistent and energetic, while simultaneously being gentle and nonviolent.

12. Incorporating visualization and breathing into your yoga practice will help you to relieve stress and any pain you might be experiencing, and to relax more deeply into difficult postures. As you inhale, visualize the breath going to the location of any pain, or visualize your breath as having the power to cause your stress to dissipate. In your mind, watch the stress melting and dissolving. It helps to have an image of your breath in the form of healing white light, and imagine it entering and leaving your body that way.

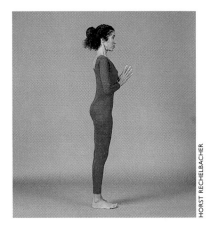

Following are some basic yoga postures that are easy to learn and include in your daily routines.

Mountain Pose

TECHNIQUE

Stand erect with your feet together, big toes touching. Contract your thighs, and tighten your kneecaps. Tuck your tailbone under; lift your spine and chest. Soften your stomach; roll your shoulders back and down; place your hands in prayer position at chest level. Keep your chin level, throat and eyes relaxed. Distribute your body weight evenly from your heels to your toes. Breathe softly and smoothly.

BENEFITS

Realigns the body, strengthens and corrects deformities of the legs, opens chest, frees and steadies the breath. Forms foundation for all other poses.

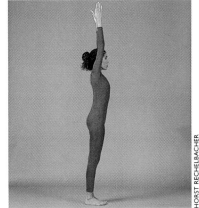

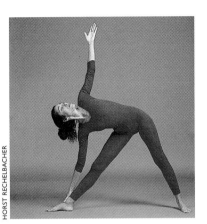

HORST RECHELBACHER

Triangle Pose

TECHNIQUE

Stand with your legs four feet apart, arms extended parallel to the floor. Turn your right foot out ninety degrees, left foot in thirty degrees, right heel in line with the middle of the left foot. Contract your thighs and tighten the kneecaps. On an exhalation, move your right hip back, and extend your trunk out over your right leg. Place your right hand on your right shin; extend your left arm straight up, palm facing forward. Keep your knees pulled up. Hold for twenty to thirty seconds. Repeat on your left side.

BENEFITS

Tones and strengthens the legs, stretches the hamstrings, opens the chest, elongates the spine.

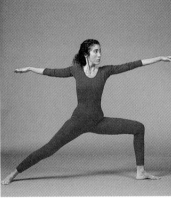

HORST RECHELBACHER

Hero Pose II

TECHNIQUE

Stand with your legs four feet apart, arms extended parallel to the floor. Turn your right foot out ninety degrees, left foot in thirty degrees, right heel in line with the middle of the left foot. Upper body maintains mountain pose. Inhale; tuck your tailbone firmly under; exhale, and bend right knee to form a right angle, keeping your left leg straight and firm. Your right knee should be in line with your right hip, directly over your right heel, shin perpendicular to the floor. Stretch your arms evenly, keeping your trunk centered over your hips. Hold for twenty to thirty seconds. Repeat on the left side.

BENEFITS

Develops stamina, strengthens ankles, knees, thighs. Stretches groin, elongates spine, opens chest, strengthens arms and back.

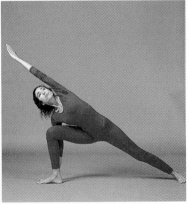

HORST RECHELBACHER

Extended Side Angle Pose

TECHNIQUE

Stand with your legs four feet apart, arms extended parallel to the floor. Turn your right foot out ninety degrees, left foot in thirty degrees, right heel in line with the middle of the left foot. Inhale; tuck your tailbone under; exhale, and bend your right knee to form a right angle. Pause. Rest your left hand on your left hip. Extend your right arm out over your right thigh, and place your hand outside your right foot. Stretch your left arm out over your left ear, palm facing the floor. Hold for twenty to thirty seconds. Repeat on the left side.

BENEFITS

Strengthens and tones legs. Reduces fat around waist and hips, elongates and stretches the spine; opens the chest. Increases movement of the bowels and aids elimination.

Camel Pose

TECHNIQUE

Kneel on the mat with your knees and feet in line with your hips. Contract your buttocks; arch your back; place your hands on your heels. Keep your pelvis pushed forward, hips over knees. Turn your toes under if the distance is too great. Drop your head back gently, keeping your neck and throat relaxed. Draw your shoulders away from your ears. Hold ten seconds; build to thirty seconds in later sessions.

BENEFITS

The whole spine is stretched and toned. Excellent for people with rounded shoulders. (Caution: People with neck problems should not do this pose without a teacher. There should be no back pain. If you cannot adjust the stretch to alleviate back pain, consult a teacher.)

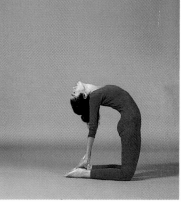

Spinal Twist

TECHNIQUE

Sit erect on the floor with your legs straight in front. Bend your right knee, and place the right foot on the floor outside the left knee. Bend the left knee, and bring the left foot outside the right hip. Turn to the right, and place your left arm as close to your shoulder as possible outside the right knee. Place your right hand on the floor as close to your back as possible, keeping the back erect. Extend your left arm and grasp your right foot with your left hand. Turn from your lower abdomen and waist, lengthening your spine upward as you turn. Hold for twenty to thirty seconds. Repeat on the left side.

BENEFITS

Tones and massages abdominal organs. Relieves back pain. Frees the movement of the shoulders.

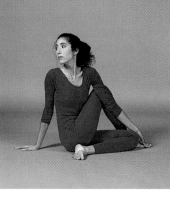

Bound Angle

TECHNIQUE

Sit erect on the floor with your legs stretched straight in front. Bend your knees, and join the soles of your feet, bringing your heels as close to the groin as possible while keeping the spine long. Wrap hands around toes, with little toes on floor. Tilt pelvis forward; descend groin; relax inner thighs. If back rounds and/or knees are higher than hips, sit on a bolster pillow high enough to drop your knees to hip level with your back straight. Hold for thirty seconds; built to two or three minutes in future sessions.

BENEFITS

Stretches inner legs; increases mobility of hips, knees, and ankles. Excellent for maintaining overall health of the pelvic organs. Together with the shoulder stand, this pose regularizes menstrual periods and helps the ovaries to function properly.

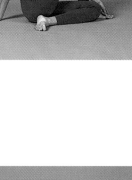

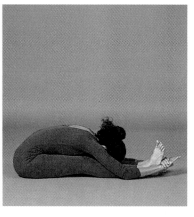

Sitting Forward Bend

TECHNIQUE

Sit erect on the floor with your legs stretched straight in front. Extend your heels; contract your thighs; tighten your kneecaps. On an exhalation, roll your pelvis forward, lift and extend your trunk out over your legs. Grasp your calves, ankles, or feet, keeping your chest open. Hold for thirty seconds; build to five minutes in future sessions. If you are stiff, sit on a rolled blanket, loop a belt around the feet, and sit erect.

BENEFITS

Stretches legs, strengthens thighs and back, stimulates and tones abdominal organs, massages the heart. Brings blood to the pelvic organs, helps to relieve impotency, and aids in control of ejaculation.

Plough Pose

TECHNIQUE

Lie on a thick blanket that elevates your shoulders and neck an inch off the floor, shoulders near the edge, neck and head off the blanket; there should be a space between your neck and the floor. Keep feet and knees together; exhale and bend your knees to your chest; then roll up onto your shoulders. Bend your elbows, and support your back with your hands. Straighten your legs, bringing your toes to the floor over your head. Contract your thighs; tighten your kneecaps; extend your heels. Lift your hips; bring the spine into your body; extend up. If your back rounds, place your feet up on a chair or wall. Do not push your chin to your chest. Hold for thirty seconds; build to three minutes in future sessions.

BENEFITS

Stretches the legs, strengthens the back. Brings flexibility to the shoulder girdle. Increases blood circulation to the neck and throat, stimulates thyroid and parathyroid glands. (Caution: Do not practice this pose during menstruation. People with neck problems should attempt this pose only under the guidance of an experienced teacher.)

Shoulder Stand

TECHNIQUE

As instructed in the plough pose, keep your feet, knees, and thighs together while bending your knees to your chest. Roll your thighs up, and extend your legs straight up to the ceiling. Tuck your tailbone under, and contract your thighs, extending your legs and back straight up. Hold for twenty to thirty seconds; build to three to five minutes in future sessions.

BENEFITS

Builds endurance, strengthens back, increases venous return to the heart, stimulates endocrine system, relieves fatigue. (Caution: Do not practice this pose during

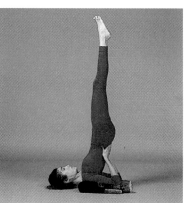

menstruation. People with neck problems or high blood pressure should attempt this pose only under the guidance of an experienced teacher.)

Headstand

TECHNIQUE

Place a folded blanket on the floor, and kneel near it. Closely interlock your fingers and rest your forearms on the blanket, elbows no wider than your shoulders. Place the crown of your head on the blanket so that the back of your head touches your palms, which are cupped. After securing your head position, raise your knees from the floor; straighten your legs; walk your toes closer to your head. Exhale, and gently lift your legs off the floor with your knees bent. Try to swing both feet off the floor simultaneously. Roll your thighs up, and straighten your legs. Lift your shoulders; tuck your tailbone under; contract your thighs. Keep your thighs, knees, and big toes touching. Do the pose against a wall if your balance is unsteady. Hold for thirty seconds; build gradually to three to five minutes in future sessions.

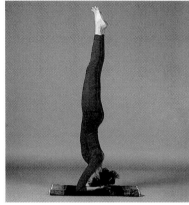

BENEFITS

Stimulates the entire organism, creates equilibrium, increases flow of blood to the brain. (Caution: Ideally, the headstand should be learned under the guidance of an experienced teacher. Also, you should become comfortable in the shoulder stand and understand its dynamics before attempting the headstand. Do not practice any inverted poses during menstruation. Do not practice the headstand if you have high blood pressure, detached retina, glaucoma, obesity, heart problems or stroke, osteoporosis, epilepsy, seizures or other brain disorders, chronic neck problems or whiplash, or conditions requiring aspirin therapy.)

Stomach Lift

TECHNIQUE

Stand with your feet in line with your hips, knees slightly bent, hands resting on your thighs. Drop your chin toward the hollow of your throat. Exhale forcefully all the air in your lungs. Holding your breath out, pull your abdominal organs toward your spine, and pull your diaphragm up, pressing your hands on your thighs. Hold for four to five seconds. Relax your abdomen; inhale slowly and smoothly. There should be no gasping. Keep your chin to your throat while relaxing your abdomen so as not to strain your heart. Take a few breaths, then repeat.

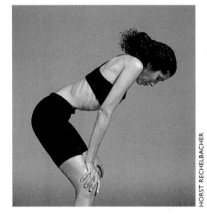

BENEFITS

Exercises and tones diaphragm and abdominal organs. Increases stomach energy, aids digestion and elimination. (Caution: Do not practice this pose if you have high blood pressure or heart problems. Practice on an empty stomach after evacuating the bladder and bowels. First thing in the morning is the best time for this pose.)

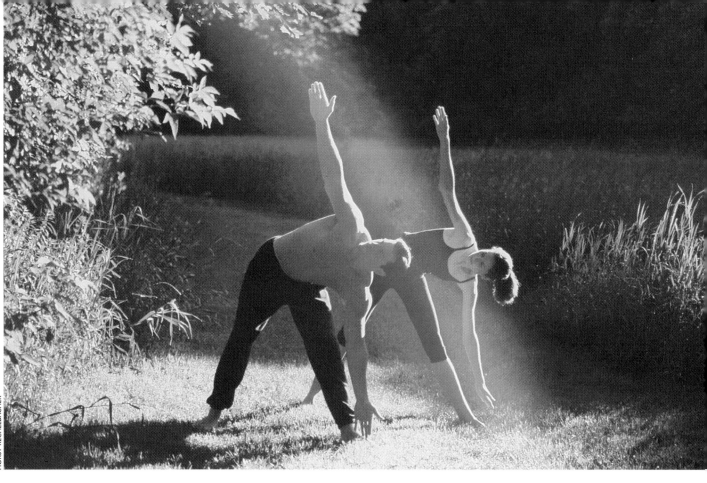

Y*oga, the mind-body-spirit workout*

Solar Salutation, or Sun Salute

The solar salutation, or sun salute, is a series of smooth movements including the poses just described. It is a routine that joins several vital poses together and encourages coordination of the breath. Before practicing this series, make sure you learn each pose separately first, familiarizing yourself with the correct positions of each. It is an excellent warm-up before any physical activity. In fact, it is a mini-yoga practice in itself when repeated three or more times. It incorporates all the necessary motions—forward bends, backward bends, groin stretches, and upper body strengtheners.

TECHNIQUE

1. Exhale, and join your palms together at the center of your chest.

2. Inhale, and stretch your arms over your head.

3. Exhale as you extend forward and down into a full forward bend. Hold for two breaths.

4. Exhale as you bend your left knee to a right angle, and stretch your right leg back, toes turned under. Knee may rest on floor if groin and/or hips are tight. Hold for two breaths.

5. Exhale, and stretch your left leg straight back, feet in line with hips and palms flat on floor. Bend your elbows in close to the sides of your chest, lower the body, and hold an inch off the floor, keeping your legs straight and your tailbone tucked. Do not arch your back. Hold for two breaths.

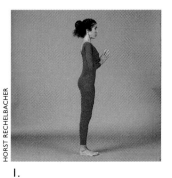

1.

6. With an exhalation, press the floor, arch your back, and lift your chest up between your arms. Stay on your toes, keeping your thighs firmly contracted and your tailbone tucked under. Hold for two breaths.

7. Exhale; lift your hips; stretch your legs back, bringing your head between your upper arms, forming an upside-down V. Stretch your spine up and your heels to the floor. Hold for two breaths.

8. Exhale, and swing your right leg forward between your hands. Keep your left leg straight back. Right knee should be over your heel, shin perpendicular to the floor. Hold for two breaths.

9. Exhale; straighten your right leg; bring your left foot next to your right to a bent-over, standing position. Knees firm, hips lifting, spine stretching down. Hold for two breaths.

10. Exhale, and stretch your arms forward and up, extending them over your head.

11. Exhale as you join your palms in the center of your chest. Hold for two breaths. This completes the cycle of the solar salutation. Repeat the entire cycle three to six times. After the last cycle, lower your arms to your sides, and align your body in the mountain pose. Remain in that pose until your breath has returned to normal.

BENEFITS

Brings flexibility to the spine and legs, stretches the chest, strengthens the arms, warms up the entire body.

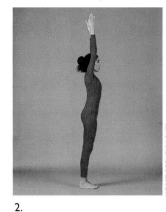

2.

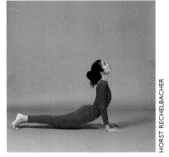

3.

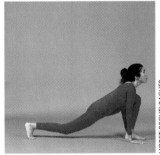

4.

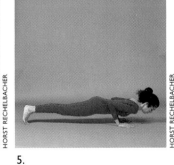

5.

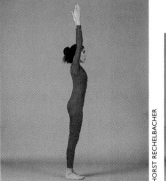

6.

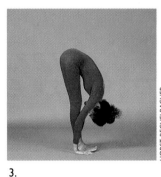

7.

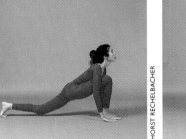

8.

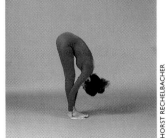

9.

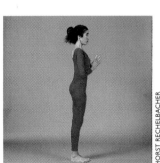

10.

11.

YOUR LIFE AS A GYM

Here are some ways to get extra exercise throughout the day:

- Park your car in a lot farther from work.
- Walk to the corner market, bank, or store rather than driving.
- Shop downtown rather than in a mall.
- Shop in a mall rather than by mail.
- Use the rest room on a different floor from your office at work.
- Take a walk over your lunch hour, or walk to meet a friend for lunch.
- Hide your remote controls.
- Wash dishes by hand.
- Walk your dog once more every day.
- Take the bus to work, and get off a stop or two earlier.
- Spend Saturday at a state park, in a museum, or on a bike ride rather than at home.
- Go out dancing (what a great excuse)!

GETTING GOING

In addition to slower modes of exercise, like yoga and some of the Asian martial arts, we should all engage in some degree of aerobic exercise each day. For some of us, the only way to get going on that sort of an exercise regimen is to join an aerobics class, go to a gym, or hire a personal trainer. Any one of these options is fine. On the other hand, lots of people exercise at home, whether they purchase cardiovascular exercise equipment, such as a cross-country skiing machine, treadmill, step machine, or stationary bicycle. Purists might invest only in a pair of walking or running shoes. Walking, running, swimming, and cycling are perfectly good aerobic choices as well, and they require minimum equipment and instruction.

In these days when most men and women work full-time, many people find the only time they have to go to the gym or to work out at home is in the evening. If it's between the evening and never, I'd say, exercise in the evening. The drawback is that aerobic exercise is invigorating, and toward the end of the day, we should be performing calming rituals to take us toward a restful sleep. A much better time for aerobic exercise is in the morning or during your lunch hour. Whenever you choose to do your more active exercise, make sure you allow for a cooling-down period, and some slow breathing to follow.

At the AVEDA plant in Blaine, Minnesota, there's a gym facility where employees can work out before or after work, or even during lunch. More and more employers are adding such facilities because they recognize that people with sound bodies are more apt to have sound minds, be healthier, and, therefore, be more productive and absent from work less frequently. It is my hope that more companies will recognize these truths and someday all workplaces will offer exercise options.

BODIES IN MOTION

There are many other forms of movement in which we can engage that we might not even think of as exercise—like gardening and dancing.

Here's a short list of some enjoyable activities that provide our bodies with different levels of motion:

- Ethnic dancing (Israeli, African, Native American, square dancing, for example) (vigorous)
- Swing dancing, disco dancing (work out at a wedding!)

▸ Gardening and weeding (moderate)
▸ Bowling (low)
▸ Massaging your partner (moderate)
▸ Walking the dog (moderate)
▸ Mowing the lawn (vigorous)

THE RIGHT AMOUNT OF EXERCISE FOR YOU

VATA EXERCISE

Type: *Amount:* light
dance aerobics
light bicycling
short hikes
walking
yoga

PITTA EXERCISE

Type: *Amount:* moderate
brisk walking or jogging
hiking
mountain climbing
skiing
swimming

KAPHA EXERCISE

Type: *Amount:* moderately heavy
aerobics
dance
rowing
running
weight training

FIT, FUN, AND PHYSICAL

Activity	Calories Burned per Hour
Fast dancing	500
In-line skating	500
Square dancing	480
Gardening	330
Playing with your kids in the park	270
Slow swimming	250
Bowling	218
Shopping (with heavy packages)	180
Kissing and hugging	135

We all have things we enjoy doing that keep us active. When you do your mirroring, think of some of the activities you like doing that give you the benefit of a workout. By incorporating more of these things into our lives, in addition to some yoga and formal exercise, we can be sure to get plenty of exercise and enjoy it at the same time. Remember, enjoying our nurturing practices is what building a nurturing life is all about.

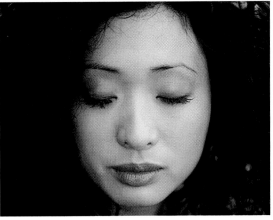

Skin Deep

Beauty is not caused. It is. —EMILY DICKINSON

Never lose an opportunity of seeing anything that is beautiful; for beauty is God's handwriting—a wayside sacrament. Welcome it in every fair face, in every fair sky, in every fair flower, and thank God for it is a cup of blessing.

—RALPH WALDO EMERSON

YOUTHFUL, HEALTHY SKIN. RADIANT BEAUTY. THESE are things we all wish for. We can achieve them—by nurturing our skin properly, by promoting a clean environment, by being as peaceful as we can be, and by getting in touch with our own individual beauty and style. In this chapter, I will help you do these things for yourself as I address the specifics of caring for the skin, shaving for men, and using makeup for women. They are all related. We need to be healthy and feel good about our complexions before we can feel good about style choices. For when we look good, we feel good, and there's no limit to what we can accomplish.

THE FACE AS A ROAD MAP

Beauty really is closely related to the health of the mind and body, and to the conditions of our surroundings. When our health is weak, when we are stressed out, or when we are exposed to too many harmful pollutants, it shows on our faces. *How* it shows can tell us a lot about what is wrong and point us toward what is causing the imbalance.

Our faces are virtual road maps to what is happening in the rest of our bodies. Some Oriental medical traditions recognized this long ago and devised systems in which the face is considered an indicator of whether a body is healthful or being weakened by disease. So it follows, then, that just as we monitor and treat the bottoms of our feet with reflexology to heal other parts of our bodies, we must also monitor our faces, and the rest of our skin, to gather clues regarding our overall well-being. We need to "listen" to our skin—look at it and know how to read what it is telling us about what is going on inside us.

Often its condition is telling us what we are eating too much or too little of. Our diet plays a big role in the condition of our skin. Naturally, it is best for us to eat foods that put very little stress on our bodies: foods that are wholesome, free of pesticides, and optimally, certified organic.

There are some foods that we know have adverse effects on the skin when they're eaten too frequently or in very high quantities. Among them are the following:

SATURATED FAT AND CHOLESTEROL: Found in meat, eggs, dairy products, poultry, and fried foods. Excessive amounts of saturated fat and cholesterol can unnaturally age the skin, making it hard, inflexible, and prone to wrinkles.

SIMPLE SUGARS: Unlike the more desirable complex carbohydrates, simple sugars give us a quick rush and then let us down. They're found in all kinds of sweets, from chocolate to cookies, and in soft drinks. They also get hidden in seemingly innocent foods like salad dressings, breads, and cereals. Simple sugars can cause capillaries near the surface of the skin to expand, creating redness and blotchiness. They can also cause body tissue to lose its natural form and consistency, making it puff and sag. On a grander scale, overconsumption of simple sugars can lead to diabetes and other blood sugar issues, raise blood pressure and triglycerides, and elevate levels of "bad" cholesterol.

SODIUM: Canned and fast foods are filled with much more sodium than we need. So are snack foods, like chips and salted nuts, and foods derived from animal sources. Sodium constricts and tightens tissue. As a result, when consumed in excessive amounts it inhibits the flow of energy. It also hardens fat and cholesterol deposits in the body. Excessive sodium may contribute to the drying, tightening, and shriveling of both skin and hair.

LOW-QUALITY LIQUIDS: The best thing we can do for our skin is drink lots of clean, purified water, about eight eight-ounce glasses a day. You can substitute some of those glasses with green tea, which combines the cleansing benefits of water with the antioxidant and anticancer effects of this miraculous tea. Drinking lots of cleansing fluid is a very simple step we can take to help our bodies perform all of their functions more smoothly and efficiently. But instead, it's not unusual for people to drink ten cups of coffee, lots of soda, beer, wine, hard liquor, milk, and juice concentrates—and drink almost no plain water. Excessive consumption of liquids, especially liquids filled with caffeine, sugar, and other toxins that the body needs to filter out, promotes a general lack of fitness, and can lead to deep horizontal lines in the forehead and bags under the eyes. It can also cause the skin to appear flabby, loose, and washed out.

PROCESSED FOODS: Modern food technology has yielded some very convenient foods of the canned, frozen, and ready-to-eat varieties. While these foods save time and often taste good, they aren't nearly as good for us as the fresh farm and garden vegetables, grains, beans, and fruits we all ate regularly before all of these innovations. Many of the nutrients in processed foods are no longer alive or active. Food without life force is inefficient nourishment that sticks to our bodies and makes them lazy. It reduces the flow of energy, makes elimination more difficult, and may contribute to a stale or wilted appearance. In contrast, whole, fresh foods possess the nutrients, life force, enzymes, and fiber necessary to help our bodies process them.

EXCESS PROTEIN: Contrary to the popular thinking of the eighties and early nineties, most adults require the same amount of protein and carbohydrates. The low-fat, high-carbohydrate diet is becoming a thing of the past, now that the medical community is recognizing that many people who adhered to that diet for years are now suffering from high cholesterol, weight gain, low energy, and blood sugar ailments such as hypoglycemia and diabetes.

On the other hand, too much protein, particularly animal-derived proteins from foods like meats, eggs, chicken, and cheese, can place tremendous stress on the kidneys and raise triglycerides. The problem is, compared to plant foods, animal proteins decompose rapidly in the body, resulting in toxic compounds such as ammonia and uric acids that accrue in the digestive system. These toxic compounds weaken the body's primary forces of elimination, the kidneys and intestines. That can lead to a toxin buildup throughout the body. An excess of animal protein can also deplete the body's calcium and mineral reserves. In addition, it can promote the accumulation of protein on the surface of the body in the form of warts, moles, calluses, and excessive body hair.

My main sources of protein are soy and fish. Soy protein helps to keep triglyceride levels low. I recommend that even nonvegetarians and big meat eaters balance their protein intake with some soy protein. The downside to eliminating animal proteins altogether is that they are a great source of B vitamins, which vegetarians often lack.

In the chapter on diet, I will address certain properties of foods and the effects they have on our bodies. I'll also discuss which foods have properties of yin, calming, and yang, stimulating, and how to incorporate both into your diet for optimal health.

Other stressors in our lives can have a huge impact on the condition of our skin. Some lifestyle factors that might be reflected on our faces are smoking, being stressed, consuming alcohol and drugs, getting too much sun, or being exposed to air pollutants. Let's just briefly take a look at each of these and see why they adversely affect our complexions:

SMOKING: The nicotine in cigarettes is a big factor in accelerated aging. It causes blood vessels to contract, preventing the normal flow of blood and nutrients to the skin's surface. Nicotine also overstimulates the nervous system, accelerating the heart rate and interfering with sleep—and who looks good without their beauty rest? Smoking has been proven to be a cause of wrinkles and loss of skin elasticity.

BEING STRESSED: Emotional stress causes certain nerves to produce proteins that trigger the immune system's white blood cells to clog the blood vessel walls. The result is sensitivity, redness, and irritation that can also lead to skin-related illnesses such as psoriasis, hives, eczema, rosacea, and acne.

CONSUMING ALCOHOL AND DRUGS: Alcohol can have a dehydrating effect on the skin. Consumed excessively, it can interfere with the liver, kidneys, and digestive system, keeping them from eliminating waste that, also, ultimately affects our skin's clarity. This can cause blood vessels to overdilate and can weaken capillary walls, drawing water out of body tissues. As a result, the skin may become dull, dry, irritated, and blotchy.

GETTING TOO MUCH SUN: In modern times, we are becoming more aware of the harmful effects of overexposure to the sun. More and more people are wearing sunscreen every day, not just when they lie out on the beach or are active in the sun. Because we are solar-powered, and because we receive vibrational nutrients as well as vitamins A and D from the sun, it is good to be in the sun about an hour a day, before the peak exposure hours of 11 A.M. to 2 P.M. in the northern hemisphere. Exposure to the sun also helps our brains to produce serotonin, which is a key to feeling happy. Too much sun exposure, resulting in sunburn or blistering, can lead to cancer down the line. The sun's ultraviolet rays can also destroy the skin's natural collagen and decrease the skin's elasticity, producing premature and extensive wrinkles. Skin that gets too much sun exposure can be dry and leathery. Don't be fooled by the lure of tanning beds as an alternative to the sun; artificial tanning is just as big a culprit in premature aging of the skin as the real sun itself.

BEING EXPOSED TO AIR POLLUTANTS: Pollution is a problem that is only getting worse. It will improve only if we all become environmentalists and activists, and avoid patronizing companies that pollute and that don't make efforts to sustain the Earth's resources. The manufacturing of synthetics and petrochemicals creates pollution in our water, soil, and air. Some of those toxins from pollution form free radicals, which deteriorate the skin—and can cause cancer. Pollution in the air equals pollution on the skin, plus dehydration. Antioxidants—taken in the form of vitamin supplements and included in our cosmetics—are our best defense against these airborne free radicals. Being an activist against corporate and private pollution is another great defense we all can take for the benefit of ourselves and the Earth's community as a whole.

Following is a listing of the parts of the body whose dis-ease might be reflected on the certain areas of the face:

INTESTINES: The forehead area can reflect imbalance of the intestines. Breakouts in this area may be an indication that the colon is congested or that purging and cleansing are occurring. If the area is red, we may be consuming too much salt, red meat, or dairy products, which are yang, or stimulating, foods. If the area is white, we may be eating too much sugar, artificial ingredients, drugs, caffeine, or fruit, which are yin, or calming, foods.

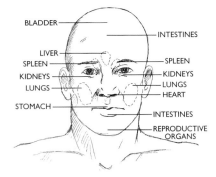

BLADDER
INTESTINES
LIVER
SPLEEN
SPLEEN
KIDNEYS
KIDNEYS
LUNGS
LUNGS
HEART
STOMACH
INTESTINES
REPRODUCTIVE ORGANS

FACIAL INDICATORS OF HEALTH AND DISEASE

LIPS: We think of digestion as taking place in the stomach, but the process really begins much sooner, at the lips. Dyes from lipstick may interfere with enzymes in the mouth and the saliva. It's a good idea to remove lipstick before eating, to aid digestion. If lips are dry and cracked, it may be a sign that the intestines are not functioning properly, or that we are eating foods too high in preservative content.

LIVER: Look between the eyes for clues to how the liver might be functioning. A vertical line here may indicate a temperamental personality. It can also be a signal of a weakness or disorder of the liver. Liver malfunctions are often caused by preservatives, alcohol and drugs, or other excessive yang substances.

SPLEEN: Lines on either side of the brow bone often indicate weakened spleen function. The spleen is another filtering organ that, once clogged with toxins, will create stress-related illnesses and changes in behavioral patterns. Lines here may also have a correlation to tightness in the shoulder area, which can be a signal that the adrenal glands are malfunctioning.

KIDNEYS: A kidney malfunction may show itself by a darkening under the eyes, either brown or black in color. If the area under the eyes is also puffy and red, we probably take in too many rich foods, alcohol, and/or nicotine or other substances with extreme yin and yang properties.

MALE REPRODUCTIVE ORGANS: Redness in the area surrounding nose may be a warning of a future malfunction of the prostate gland. Redness may also suggest that we are eating too many foods that have extreme yang properties. Whiteness in this area can be an indication that we are eating too many foods with extreme yin properties.

HEART: Redness, expanded capillaries, or swollen tissue at the tip of the nose may indicate high blood pressure and a tendency toward heart conditions.

LUNGS: If there are blackheads, whiteheads, or irritations in the nostrils and cheek area, we probably have frequent colds and bronchitis and consume a fair amount of dairy products, which form mucus in the lungs, as well as sugar, a food with extreme yin.

STOMACH: Breakouts in the area surrounding the lips may indicate an inability to digest food well, possibly due to an enzyme deficiency in the acid of the stomach.

FEMALE REPRODUCTIVE ORGANS: Breakouts in the chin area are usually related to the menstrual cycle. Areas on the sides of the chin that are white and blotchy, either with congestion or suffocation, resulting in a small granular-like feeling under the skin, may indicate a yeast infection. If the chin is always red, swollen, and either suffocated or congested, it may mean that there is some structural weakness of the reproductive organs.

All of these ailments can be counteracted with a combination of proper diet, exercise, daily skin care, and peacefulness of mind, body, and spirit. In fact, a clear, healthy complexion is one of the great incentives for us to design a routine of nurturing daily practices.

ONE DAY AT A TIME

Each day is a new opportunity to treat ourselves well, and with regard to our skin, it is a chance to enhance our beauty and preserve it from the harmful effects of the elements. When we create a day-long routine of nurturing practices addressing all the aspects of our lives, we must include those specifically aimed at skin care. Start these with morning cleansing, toning, moisturizing and making up; and end with an evening habit of cleansing, toning, and moisturizing.

Actually, it doesn't really end there. The things we do all day, the emotions we have, and the foods we eat are also related to our skin care, and will even affect our complexion while we sleep. Also, our self–face massage each morning promotes the emission of toxins from glands in the face and stimulates circulation. The yoga postures we do that require inversion, such as headstands and shoulder stands, also help our complexion by increasing blood flow and the distribution of nutrients in the blood to the face.

Taking care of our skin is a combination of nurturance and defense. We must feed and clean our skin, but we must also protect it from harmful things in the environment, including the sun and free radicals, which are ions derived from ultraviolet rays and pollution that break down the skin's natural supply of collagen and elastin. Every day, our skin is under attack from the damaging effects of dirt, dust, air pollution, the sun, and the drying wind. There are three steps which we can take, twice a day, to counteract those effects: cleansing, nourishing, and toning our skin. Let's look at each of these in depth.

Cleansing

Regardless of how simple or elaborate our daily routines of skin care have been, we all know about the importance of removing dirt, oil, and dry flakes from our skin. We all wash our faces. But we don't all use the best cleansing products for our skin. It is important to use cleansers that are natural and have an alkaline base. These cleansers can help to clean pores very deeply. They also don't put stress on the cells, unlike acid-based synthetic cleansers, which tighten pores, straining the skin. Cleansers are available in gel or cream form. Gel cleansers have a foaming effect and are preferred for oily skin; cream cleansers lubricate as they remove dirt and are recommended for dry skin.

Whichever form of cleanser you choose, you want to make sure that your facial wash contains essential oils because essential oils are solvents by nature. They dissolve waxes and impurities and help remove them from your skin. Essential oils are also natural antiseptics, which fight the bacteria that cause acne and other blemishes. Scrubbing your face with a facial cleanser that contains active essential oils will allow you to get in deep, stimulate the skin, and promote exfoliation.

A facial scrub, with natural granules of some sort, is an excellent daily cleansing substance. It helps to exfoliate the skin, which is necessary in order to avoid the clogging of pores, by removing the top layer of dead skin. This daily stimulation of your skin will help you maintain a healthy, youthful complexion.

Washing and scrubbing should both include a gentle massage that works over all parts of your face in a circular motion. The water you're using should be neither too hot nor too cold. Move your fingers upward and outward in circles, and avoid getting too close to the eye area. After you have cleaned and rinsed your face, don't wipe it dry—pat it gently with a clean towel.

After cleansing, it is a good idea to use an exfoliant with alpha- and beta-hydroxies. This will be a clear, astringent liquid that will loosen dead skin so that the next time you do your cleansing, exfoliation will be easier.

On days when you don't use an exfoliant, I recommend using an astringent toner—something as simple as rose water—to close the pores and keep them from absorbing new dirt and oil.

Toning

The second step in our twice-daily skin regimen should be toning. Most toners are astringents that help remove whatever impurities are left after

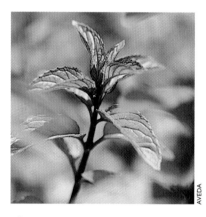

A mint spritz can tone and refresh your complexion any time and cool your skin in the heat of summer.

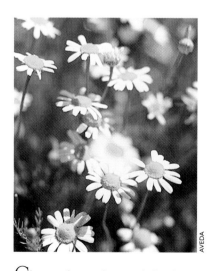

Chamomile, gentle enough for the most sensitive skin

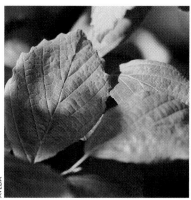

AVEDA

Witch hazel has long been used as a natural astringent toner.

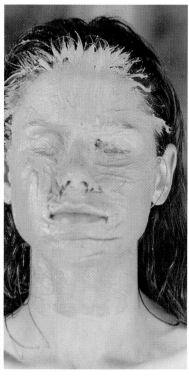

HORST RECHELBACHER

Avocado makes a most nourishing masque.

cleansing, and that help close the pores so that new impurities we might encounter won't have an open hole in which to hide. The most effective toners are those made from flower essences. Rose water and witch hazel both have long histories as facial toners. Rose water has been used through the ages and is made by soaking rose petals for many days in distilled water. The rose water has yin, or cooling and relaxing qualities. You may add other essences to rose water, to create a new toner, tailored to your individual skin type. Apply the toner of your choice in a light spray, making sure your eyes are closed. After that, use your dry fingers to press the moisture into your skin. Follow this with a moisturizer.

Nourishing

We can feed our skin two types of nourishment: masques and moisturizers. Both are lovely additions to our daily skin care routine.

Masques are not used as regularly as moisturizers by many, but you should consider their benefits and include them more often in your daily regimen. Aside from their obvious nurturing qualities for our skin, masques give us a chance to take some time to relax since we must leave them on for a period of five to fifteen minutes to work their magic. There are different types of masques. There are deep-cleansing masques that open and cleanse the pores, which you can employ at the beginning of your skin-cleansing routine, and nourishing masques that fortify the skin with restorative nutrients, which you can use at the end of your routine. Both of these types of masques should be used about once a week. You may want to steam your face over a basin of hot water and essential oils to open up your pores before applying a cleansing masque.

There are masques with heating effects that stimulate the circulation of blood at the surface of the skin (yang), and those that have a relaxing and cooling effect (yin), and contract the pores and facial blood vessels. Both types of masques can be used in succession, beginning with a stimulating masque. When we don't have time to use both masques in one sitting, we can use a stimulating masque in the morning, to help us get going for the day, and a relaxing masque in the evening, when we're ready to unwind.

It is important to make sure our masques are made with nourishing infusions that suit our skin types. We need to stabilize our skin and its natural oils. There are infusions that are best for oily, normal, dry, and combination skin. On the facing page is a list of skin conditions and skin types and the essences that are good for them. Remember, always buy or prepare a masque

NATURE'S ANSWER TO YOUR SKIN

DRY SKIN	ESSENTIAL OIL		
Chapped skin	Chamomile	Myrrh	Rose
	Lavender	Palmarosa	Sandalwood
Dermatitis	Chamomile	Lavender	

OILY SKIN/ACNE	ESSENTIAL OIL		
Blemished	Bergamot	Grapefruit	Patchouli
	Chamomile	Juniper berry	Peppermint
	Clary sage	Lavender	Rosemary
	Cypress	Lemon	Tea tree
	Eucalyptus	Orange	
Seborrhea	Bergamot	Orange	Sandalwood
	Cypress	Patchouli	Tea tree
	Geranium	Rosemary	Ylang-ylang
	Lavender	Sage	
Blackheads	Bergamot	Geranium	
	Cedarwood	Lavender	

SENSITIVE SKIN	ESSENTIAL OIL		
	Chamomile	Lavender	Rose
	Geranium	Neroli	

AGING SKIN	ESSENTIAL OIL		
Dehydration	Chamomile	Lavender	Sandalwood
	Cypress	Myrrh	Palmarosa
	Geranium	Neroli	
	Jasmine	Rose	
Sagging skin	Bergamot	Lavender	

NORMAL/COMBINATION SKIN	ESSENTIAL OIL		
	Bergamot	Lavender	Ylang-ylang
	Jasmine	Rose	

SPECIAL SKIN CONDITIONS	ESSENTIAL OIL		
Cellulite	Basil	Juniper	Rose
	Cedar	Neroli	Rosemary
	Fennel	Orange	Tea tree
	Geranium	Patchouli	
Stretch marks	Geranium	Neroli	Patchouli
	Lavender	Olibanum	Rose
Thread veins	Chamomile	Geranium	
	Cypress	Lavender	

with these oils; never apply oils directly to your skin. They are too concentrated and can burn or irritate your skin badly if used alone.

Moisturizers are the second form of skin nourishment, and they should also be chosen to suit our skin types. We all need a moisturizer, no matter how naturally oily our skin may be. Moisturizer pleases the skin. In fact, not moisturizing oily skin can lead to pimples. When oily skin isn't kept moist on the surface, the top layer gets dry and contracts, trapping oil and bacteria underneath, leading to skin eruptions. The market is now filled with oil-free moisturizers for those who have oily skin. AVEDA makes a product, called Oil-Free Hydraderm, which contains mainly oil-free, natural aloe vera. There are lots of moisturizers that do contain oil, but natural oils which are easily assimilated into the skin. Whatever moisturizer you choose, bear in mind that one with a high concentration of natural ingredients, and a low level of petrochemicals, will be best for the health and appearance of your skin.

There are also many moisturizers available with sun protection factors (SPFs), now that we're all so aware of the damaging effects of the sun and the rapid thinning of the Earth's protective ozone layer. Those of us who do not wear foundation makeup—and these are available with SPFs, too—should definitely look for moisturizers that protect skin from the sun. We all have to protect ourselves every day from the sun's rays, not just when we hit the beaches in June, July, and August.

Moisturizers these days are also available with plenty of antioxidants, which are very helpful in counteracting the effects of free radicals. Vitamins A, C, D, and E have antioxidant properties. Moisturizers that contain these and other antioxidants will help us to remain young-looking by protecting our skin from those substances in our environment that break down the collagen and elastin in our skin.

After toning and cleansing, apply moisturizer gently to the skin, avoiding the eye areas. Press into the skin gently.

WHAT'S MY TYPE?

How we treat our skin should be determined by our skin type. Most of us are probably aware of whether we have normal, dry, oily, acne-prone, or combination skin, but maybe we don't know exactly what products are best for our type of complexion.

I have compiled a basic guide that helps my clients at AVEDA determine and treat each skin type. These guidelines apply to both men and women. More men today are taking mindful care of their skin than in the past, as well they should. After all, men are exposed to the same elements as women—and, in addition, most men don't have the additional protection of a layer of makeup that women do to shield them from the environmental factors of dirt and sun.

Dry Skin

Dry skin, obviously, is low on moisture. It also tends to be thinner than normal skin, and to show expanded capillaries and blemishes from sensitivity. This can make dry skin look red and blotchy. The pores on the nose, forehead, and chin often are larger than those in other areas. When skin eruptions do appear, they are usually in the form of whiteheads, filled with sebum, the body's natural oil. This oil is stuck because it can't escape through the contracted pores of the skin's dry surface layer. These are some tips that will aid in keeping dry skin moist and clear.

> Wash at least once daily with a cream cleanser that helps remove the sebum from beneath the skin without drying it out. Avoid foaming cleansers.

> Stimulate the skin, such as by massaging, to help remove the oil. But keep the stimulation moderate for dry skin, as it is easily irritated by too much rubbing.

> Avoid harsh chemicals and potent formulas.

> Use a cleansing scrub once or twice a week. Slow and gentle circular motions will keep the scrub from being too abrasive to the skin.

> Facial masques should have moisturizing properties, to replenish the skin, keep it moist and plump and help to rid the skin of embedded particles such as blackheads and whiteheads.

> Help neutralize the skin and bring the moisture further into the skin with a rose water facial toner after a masque.

> Keep the skin hydrated and protected with a rich moisturizer.

Oily Skin

There are positive and negative aspects to having oily skin. Oily skin is smoother in texture, and thicker and more pliable than dry skin because it retains more sebum. That sebum might keep skin from heavy wrinkling, but it also leads to blackheads, pustules (or blackheads that have broken through the skin's surface and become infected), and whiteheads. So, while those with oily skin tend to remain youthful-looking longer, they must guard against a greasy look and take steps to prevent skin breakouts and acne.

While one's inclination with oily skin might be to wash and wash, and scrub and scrub, this can actually have the adverse effect of making the skin secrete even more oil. The best weapons against highly oily skin are eating a healthy diet, aimed at reducing oil secretion, and using natural skin products that cleanse but don't overstimulate the skin. Here are some other pointers those with this skin type may find helpful:

▹ Cleanse two to three times daily, using a foaming cleanser at least one of those times. Cream cleansers can also be used.

▹ Don't overclean. Overcleansing will lead only to the secretion of even more oil.

▹ Use a natural cleansing scrub once a week to remove eruptions and to stimulate the purging of particles from beneath the skin's surface.

▹ Nourish, moisturize, soften, tone, and tighten the skin with a stimulating (yang) masque.

▹ Help purge, cleanse, and moisturize the skin and normalize sebum production with a relaxing (yin) masque. Remember, even the oiliest skin needs to be moisturized.

▹ Neutralize the skin and prepare it to receive moisture with a gentler toner.

▹ Use an oil-free moisturizer, which is probably best for oily skin. They are usually made of plant matter, such as aloe vera, and promote softness without greasiness.

Combination Skin

People with combination skin have characteristics of both oily and dry skin, in different areas of their faces. Make note of the areas that you find oily and those that seem dry. Refer to information earlier in this chapter on those areas of the face and the body systems that might correspond with them. Review your diet and consider how proper eating can restore balance in your skin and follow the guidelines above, for oily and dry skin, for treating those areas.

Normal Skin

People with normal skin rarely have eruptions on the face, and when they do, they're usually due to stress, climate changes, hormonal disturbances, or alterations in nutrition. Their skin color is usually pretty even, and the skin typically has a "healthy glow" and plenty of moisture. As wonderful as this skin type is, even those of us who are blessed with normal skin must care for it properly in order to maintain that healthy glow. Here are some suggestions:

⟩ Use a cleansing cream for normal to dry skin twice a day to remove impurities and excess oil.

⟩ Help remove built-up oil and keep the blood and nutrients flowing through the skin with twice-daily stimulation, through circular, massaging motions.

⟩ Exfoliate regularly with a natural cleansing scrub.

⟩ Neutralize the skin's surface with a natural facial toner.

⟩ Hydrate the skin and seal in moisture using a moisturizer with or without oil.

A CLEAN SHAVE

Although men are becoming more aware of the importance of skin care, most men still have a long way to go to incorporate a nurturing skin care routine to their day. For example, not many men recognize shaving as an important part of their skin care regimen. In fact, most men probably don't give shaving much thought at all. They just do it and get it over with, stoically enduring frequent nicks and cuts. But shaving does more than just remove facial hair. It also helps to exfoliate the skin, lifting dead skin cells from the surface. This creates a smoother surface and healthier skin. When we use shaving products that are natural and that contain essential oils, the benefits to our skin are even greater. Shaving needs to be reconsidered and understood by men as one of their nurturing daily habits. Here are some tips for making it a more positive experience.

⟩ Spend more than three minutes shaving. Take your time. Haste often makes stinging cuts.

⟩ On the face, always shave in one direction, either with or against the hair's natural growth. Do not vary. Choose one way or the other and stick with it. Otherwise, you'll experience discomfort and irritation.

⟩ On the neck, where hair grows in various directions, it's all right to shave in different directions. But go over each section only once.

⟩ If you experience ingrown hairs, you may be shaving the same area twice, or shaving too closely.

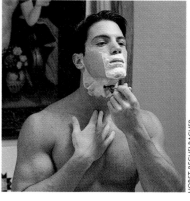

*T*ake a little time; start your day with a meditative shave.

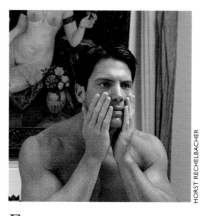

*E*ssential oils enhance the shaving experience.

AFTERSHAVE OPTIONS

You can easily create your own aftershave by using essential oils in combination with alcohol and a base oil such as jojoba oil, wheat germ oil, almond oil, or hemp oil. Here's a basic guide to some of the oils and their scent types:

▸ *Spicy/musky scents:*

cinnamon, cassia, caraway, cardamom, pepper, olibanum, myrrh, cypress, sage, patchouli

▸ *Light citrusy scents:*

bergamot, lemon, lime, orange

▸ Use an exfoliant on your skin at night; this can be helpful toward avoiding ingrown hairs. It helps to loosen the ends of the hair that can get stuck in the skin.

Shaving can actually be quite meditative and satisfying spiritually, especially if you bring pleasing aromatics into the shaving ritual by using essential oils as an aftershave. Men of different generations and backgrounds will respond to different types of scents. Right now, the lemon and lime scents that were popular in the fifties are making comeback. Musks were popular in the sixties and seventies, and are still popular with people who first started wearing aftershave then. But above all, the best scents to choose are the ones to which you personally respond.

THE EYE OF THE BEHOLDER

Making ourselves as beautiful as we can be is a process that we all approach from without and from within. We each have our own unique brand of beauty, which is reflected from the inside out. Beauty exists in every one of us, but it needs to be discovered. We all have a tendency to adopt the aesthetic ideals of the people around us, and those put forth by magazines, before really even considering our own ideas about style, and our individual beauty. From the time that we are teenagers, we seek the input and approval of peers. This is a natural impulse. However, it is important also to add our own personal touches to our makeup, hair, and overall style. Some women who learned to put on makeup when they were fourteen still apply it the way an older sibling or friend taught them. They haven't updated their approach, or figured out a way to do their makeup that suits their features best. Discovering our own signature beauty and style can be a very exciting journey, as we examine ourselves inside and out. It requires mirroring, taking inventory of our own ideas, our strengths, and those things that we would like to accentuate.

We all have the potential to enhance our beauty. It begins with a daily practice of self-awakening, self-realization, and self-appreciation. For once, in the privacy of our own mirroring sessions, let's not be modest! Admit to ourselves what we like about our looks, about our expressions, about our bodies. Before crafting a personal style—with or without the help of a professional stylist or makeup artist—I recommend taking a personal inventory of the things you'd like to accentuate about your features, and the things from which you'd like to draw attention away. Divide a piece of paper in half, and begin with the things you're fond of. Try not to be modest. Allow yourself to like what you see in yourself.

Those things you want to stand out can be accentuated with makeup. Before we make changes in our beauty routines, it's a good idea to have a makeover, or a makeup lesson. These are usually very valuable sessions with an experienced makeup artist who can inform you of current trends in beauty, as well as general, timeless, effective techniques. I actually recommend getting a makeup lesson or makeover two or three times a year. These can be pampering experiences and also very informative ones. They are not frivolous, either. In the world today, looking current, polished, and well put together is an important component of success.

When you go for a makeup lesson, choose a company like AVEDA, whose makeup products are as natural as possible. Makeup with pure emollients and protective plant and mineral ingredients actually nurtures the skin, acting as a very healthy element of your skin care routine. This is most important for the health and appearance of our skin.

Makeup with a high concentration of petrochemical ingredients is bad for our skin—and our environment. Many of the synthetics used in many makeup lines can be cancer-causing. They put stress on our cells because they are foreign to our cells, and that can promote premature aging. In addition, many of those synthetics are not biodegradable, which means they exist in our midst and pollute the Earth indefinitely. It's also a good idea to find a company that offers recyclable/reusable makeup containers, for the benefit of the Earth and everyone who lives here.

When choosing a makeup artist to learn from, try to choose someone who seems to have a personal style similar to yours, or that which you want to adopt. That way you'll know that person will be attuned to your taste and desires, and will help you zero in on the look you want to create for yourself.

INTO THE WOODS

One of the greatest learning experiences of my life has been going to the rain forest in South America, first with the late Deborah "Moonstar" Rinkel, and, since 1992, with ethnobotanist May Waddington, an important source for AVEDA in that region of the world. In my travels to the rain forest, I have learned so much about natural, sustainable plant sources for color, such as uruku, and about how other people live, particularly the indigenous Yawanawa tribe living in Nova Esperanca, a remote western town of Brazil.

COLOR COORDINATED

Here are some current color concepts to keep in mind when trying new makeup techniques on yourself:

▸ Moonlights—How can you look dramatic without redoing the same old evening look? Let moonlight and stardust seep over your entire face—lids, lips, and cheeks—with sheer washes of shimmer over more traditional makeup.

▸ Painted nudes—The new face is more about luminous skin than come-lately colors. You know the drill—sleep, exercise, and plenty of water. Until hard work pays off, fake it with foundation or cream concealer applied only where needed. Once you've earned your healthy glow, you'll need just a light dusting of loose powder (and a personal water cooler).

▸ All and nothing—Recent bolder hues are more fun than we've had in years. But as with all good things, enjoy in moderation. Taking more than one feature into full color can be overkill. Be truly modern by wearing the rest of your face boldly bare while making a fashion statement by accentuating your mouth, or your eyes—but remember, accentuate *just one thing.*

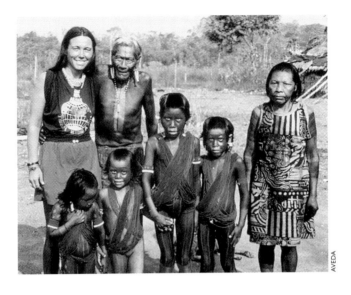

AVEDA

A Yawanawa shaman and his family with AVEDA's herbalist, Moonstar.

Since 1993, AVEDA has been involved in a partnership with the Yawanawa. There, the tribe grows the uruku tree, which provides natural plant pigment used in AVEDA products. For the Yawanawa, our arrangement provides a measure of economic independence.

I traveled with May Waddington to Nova Esperanca in 1993 to meet with the leaders of sixteen indigenous tribes to explore partnership possibilities. AVEDA's research chemists had discovered that the uruku, or Bixa orellana plant, contained a pigment that was ideal for creating lipstick color. The uruku is a bushy tree that grows to a height of about nine feet and produces red or green pods that contain deep orange, pigment-bearing seeds which have been used for centuries by the Yawanawa and other tribes to color their faces and bodies for ceremonies. It is also used in the form of colorau, a bright orange, paprika-like powder used in cooking by combining the ground uruku seeds with manioc, a starchy root that's a staple in the Brazilian diet.

May recommended working with Biraci Brasil (known as Bira), the chief of the Yawanawa tribe. He had been a friend of May's from her days working in the indigenous rights movement there.

For those for whom the word *chief* conjures images of stern old men with creased faces, Bira comes as a surprise. In his early thirties and with a penchant for bright-colored T-shirts, rubber flip-flops, and fierce games of pick-up volleyball, he looks more like a resident of Miami Beach or L.A. But most striking about Bira are his powerful sense of spirituality and purpose, and his profound awareness of the challenges facing his tribe. Foremost among these is reclaiming the Yawanawa culture, which was nearly erased by decades of domination by rubber barons and missionaries.

According to Bira, the Yawanawa people are part of the Pano linguistic group, descended from the Inca ancestors who migrated from the Andes to western Brazil centuries ago. Though the tribe was legendary for never being dominated by others, by the time Bira was born, white rubber barons and missionaries were well established in the Yawanawa village—dictating a new tone for economic and religious life for the entire tribe. When the Yawanawa worked as rubber trappers, most of the profits went to the bosses. During the thirty years the missionaries held sway, almost 80 percent of the tribe converted to their very strict form of Protestantism, which frowned on traditional Yawanawa rituals and forbade many tribal customs, including polygamy (a custom that is still being practiced in Nova Esperanca and other parts of the world today).

As a young man, Bira was chosen by the missionaries to join their calling and was sent to the small city of Rio Branco to study. There, he discovered that laws existed that guaranteed the rights of indigenous peoples, and there was even a government agency to oversee indigenous affairs. The missionaries had hidden this information from the Yawanawa. Bira returned to his hometown with this knowledge and led the Yawanawa in a fight to reclaim their land. They succeeded in 1984 when their traditional area was demarcated by the Brazilian government.

Although they won the battle, the war persists, even today. The Yawanawa continue to face many of the same issues: missionaries remain a divisive presence in the area; outsiders still want the land for their own economic gain.

However, the Yawanawa are now better able to resist this interference because of the economic independence they have achieved through their partnership with AVEDA. For Bira, this foray into the modern economy is a tool that will help the tribe to live as it chooses. His plan for the tribe is to operate as an independent business with outside interests like AVEDA to achieve its goals.

"We want to develop into a microcompany," Bira says, "a company that processes uruku, that researches uses for the hundreds of trees that grow here, that manufactures plant oils to offer the world for cosmetic use." Bira sees the Yawanawa becoming a "modern tribe"—a people who utilize the resources of the modern world to enable them to live in harmony with their land and traditions.

AVEDA currently uses uruku grown at the village in three Uruku Lip Colours, three Uruku Lip Sheers, and Bixa and Annato Colour Conditioners. Our research chemists are currently working on ways to utilize the pigment in more products, including shampoo and permanent hair color.

On a recent visit to the village, May brought along some of AVEDA's uruku products so the tribe could see the end result of their work. One man remarked that he was proud his work had resulted in something so beautiful.

AVEDA is working now with some other tribes to explore the possibilities of a mutually beneficial partnership for harvesting plants for natural pigments and nutritional use. Among these tribes are the Caiua, Guarani, and Terena peoples who share a reservation in central Brazil. Convinced twenty years ago to cut down their noble woods with the promise that all would receive a house in return, the tribes deforested their land with their own hands—but the promise was never kept. Now the land is as clear as a midwestern prairie, and the people have been left with nothing: no birds, no game, no wood for burning or building, no houses. It is a situation made all the more tragic by the fact that they live right next to a wealthy boomtown built in large part by the exploitation of their land by others. For many, their only income comes from leasing their land to outside farmers, whose use of petrochemical fertilizers and herbicides compromised the health of the land as well as that of the people who live on it. Their plight has led to a high rate of suicide on the reservation.

Tribes like these need autonomy, and they need the resources to make autonomy possible. "We need allies like AVEDA, who come from other cities to listen to the people," says Bira, who is well acquainted with the plight of other tribes like the Caiua. "We're looking for our own alternatives. AVEDA sees this partnership not as a handout but as respect for the community and for nature. This is an example that can give fruit—the fact that there's support for our little group in the rain forest from a big company in the United States. This is an example of dignity." And true beauty.

MAKEUP ABC'S

For those of us who don't have the option of going to a professional makeup artist, the following is a basic guide to applying makeup. We can each adjust these guidelines to fit our personal likes and dislikes.

Complexion

▸ Make time to think about how you want to look, and to try different looks. Don't feel guilty about the time it takes to do this. This investment of time, energy, and focus is part of treating yourself well and creating total harmony between your inner and outer being.

▸ Apply makeup with good, natural-hair brushes, which are better than the little applicators that come with the products.

▸ Use a concealer that's lighter than your skin to help conceal bags under your eyes and any blemishes. Blend it in with a back-and-forth, patting motion. Don't use too much—less is often more where makeup application is concerned!

▸ Never cover open abrasions with concealer; this can lead to infection.

▸ If you've never worn foundation, consider adding it to your makeup regimen as a protectant. A lightweight foundation with antioxidants and SPFs can be a great shield against the sun, wind, and free radicals. The opaqueness of foundation makes it a better sun block than a moisturizer with SPFs.

▶ Choose a foundation that is right for your skin type and skin color. If you have oily skin, try to find an oil-free foundation. Choose a color that closely matches your skin, so that it is virtually imperceptible, or slightly darker than your complexion. But also be flexible and remember to change foundation colors with the seasons, as your skin tone varies.

▶ Apply foundation either with the fingers or a sponge. A sponge gives a more natural, sheerer application. After the foundation is applied, blend it downward, gently, into the skin.

▶ Find a pressed powder that is a bit lighter than your foundation, so the skin doesn't look dirty after you apply it. Pressed powder gives a finished, matte look to the makeup. Too much, though, and the skin looks cakey. So apply this layer sparingly.

▶ Use a powder puff to press and roll the powder onto the face evenly.

Eyes

The eyes are the "windows of the soul," many believe. They are also most people's favorite feature on themselves. Many people like to accentuate the eyes, although there are those who believe the eyes stand out on their own and don't need any help. For those who want to accentuate, here are some tips:

▶ Choose an eyeliner that is made without harmful preservatives, and which contains antioxidants like vitamin E. Pick a color that complements your eye color. Some people like to choose colors opposite to their eye color. You can also accentuate the color you have with a different shade of it. There are no rules. It all depends on whether you want to accentuate or downplay your eyes. Highlight with contrasting colors; downplay with similar colors. And use your own fashion sense.

▶ Apply the pencil at the lash line, and then soften it by blending carefully with a brush.

▶ Set the eyeliner in place by gently tapping a loose powder on the closed eye. The loose powder should match your skin tone of either yellow or pink.

▶ Choose two colors of eye shadow—a light neutral and a darker contour color. Shadows enhanced with antioxidants like vitamins A, C, and E will help to promote youthful, healthier-looking skin around your eyes.

▶ Apply the neutral shadow over the entire eye area, going above the crease. Blend well.

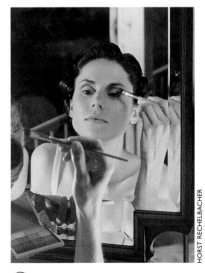

Give eyes a boost of color and nutrients with shadows that nurture skin with vitamins A, C, and E.

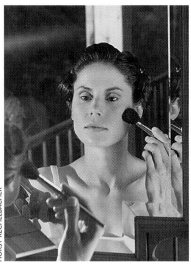

Get that sunkissed look with a blush that emulates your natural one after a day at the beach.

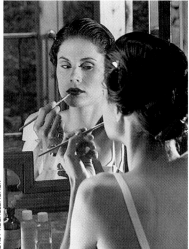

Your lip colors probably look good— but do they taste good? They should!

▸ Apply the darker contour color at the lash line, blending upward and outward.

▸ Choose a natural mascara to thicken and lengthen lashes. Pick a color that looks natural on you. Brown can be less stark than black on people with light hair.

▸ Apply the mascara to the upper and lower lashes, gently stroking upward and outward from roots to tips. As you do so, twist the wand to lift and curl the lashes.

▸ Fill in the eyebrows, too, with eye shadow that closely matches the color of the brow. Go easy here. You don't want to make your eyebrows look too heavy. You can use pencils, too, but shadows look more natural.

Cheeks

Wouldn't it be great if we could always be naturally tanned and rosy-cheeked? The next best thing is a natural-toned blush, in a pink-brown base that looks like the color of skin when it naturally tans.

▸ Choose a blush that has naturally derived ingredients and antioxidants, in a color that matches the skin's natural radiance.

▸ Apply lightly with a brush, sponge, or powder puff in a circular motion from the apple of the cheek toward the hairline.

▸ If you accidentally applied too much blush, use more pressed powder to tone it down.

Lips

Lip color is the simplest way to change your entire look. It's an easy way to pull your whole face together and appear made-up, even if you're not. Lip color is also a great way to protect lips—provided you use lip pencils, lipsticks, and glosses that are free of carcinogens, and that contain antioxidants.

When you're choosing a lipstick, it is very important to pay attention not only to the color and texture, but to the ingredients as well. If you were to bring a magnifying glass to the cosmetics counter or the drugstore to read the fine-printed list of ingredients on most lipsticks, you'd find a good number of indigestible petrochemical waxes that can be quite harmful in high dosages. The skin on our lips is much thinner than that on the rest of the face, and so the chemicals in lipsticks are very easily absorbed into our bodies and our bloodstreams. In addition, considering that lipstick is situated at the entrance to your mouth, you wind up eating quite a bit of it over time. Did you ever stop to consider how many pounds of lipstick you will eat in your lifetime? Better to choose lipsticks, like AVEDA's, that are filled with ingredients which are actually good for you. I have always tried to make lipsticks that have health benefits, with ingredients like beeswax, calendula, and other plant waxes; essential oils such as basil, peppermint, anise, and fennel; and antioxidants such as vitamin E.

Here are some other lip tips:

▹ Use lip pencil when a more defined lip is desired. Lip pencil will also lengthen the wear of your lipstick, help prevent lipstick from feathering beyond the lip line, and can be used alone for a matte look.

▹ Sharpen your lip pencil before using it to ensure a clean tip.

▹ Choose a color that coordinates closely with the lip color you've chosen.

▹ Follow the natural contour of your lips.

▹ Fill in entire mouth with the lip pencil for greater color consistency and longevity.

▹ Apply lip color—lipstick or gloss—liberally over entire mouth with a lip brush for greater control. Fill the center of the lips in first, then perfect the outer edges.

▹ Choose which look you want to go with—more natural or highly glamorous—and plan your makeup accordingly. Makeup that's good for your skin can be subtle or very dramatic in its tones and effects.

Remember, in the morning it's a good idea to wait to apply lipstick until after breakfast is finished.

Now it's time to style your hair. You'll find lots of hair care and styling tips ahead in the next chapter.

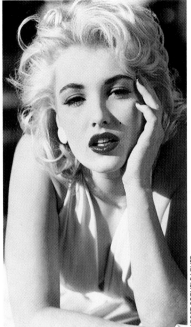

HORST RECHELBACHER

*H*ollywood high style

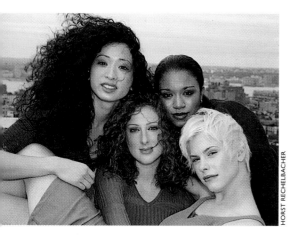

HORST RECHELBACHER

Good Hair Days

The body is the shell of the soul, and dress the husk of that shell; but the husk often tells what the kernel is.

—ANONYMOUS

WE ALL HAVE OUR SHARE OF GOOD AND BAD HAIR days. In the grander scheme of things, when we're talking about spiritual contentment and global consciousness, it might seem superficial to concern ourselves with the appearance of our tresses. But as anyone who has ever had a bad hair day knows, this phenomenon, like so many others, is only one part physical.

There are emotional and spiritual factors that affect, and result from, our outward presentation. For me, a bad hair day usually begins before I've done anything to my hair. It has to do with my state of being, related to other people, conditions, and events that affect my life. My health makes a difference. If I don't feel good about the way I look, and I don't like the style, color, or texture of my hair, chances are I'm not going to feel confident facing the world.

The same is true of good hair days. When everything seems right, chances are I will be more apt to look good, and put more energy into grooming. When we're happy and glowing, it almost doesn't matter if a few strands of hair are out of place, or if that stubborn cowlick is standing up again. Our radiance overshadows any of the very imperfections on which we might fixate during a bad hair day. Yet good hairstyling itself can be the launch of a good day. Feeling positive about our appearance often helps us to feel positive in other areas of our lives.

After all, our hair says a lot about us. The way we wear it—the cut and style we choose—says quite a bit about our aesthetics, and how we feel about ourselves. Furthermore, the condition of our hair reflects what is going on inside of us, as well as how we care for ourselves. But basic, beautiful, healthy, chic hair can be a reality for everyone. All it requires is some attention, the adjustment of a few details in our daily routines, and a good stylist.

Cleaning and styling our hair regularly is not likely to be a new practice for anyone reading this book. It's something most of us do every day without even thinking. But now we should do some thinking about this particular set of rituals, how we go about it, and the products that we use. In this chapter, I'll talk about cleaning, conditioning, styling, and coloring hair in ways that are nurturing not only to each strand of hair on our heads, but to our psyches and all the cells of our bodies as well.

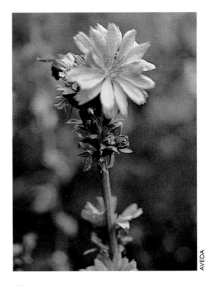

Blue malva naturally heightens highlights in all hair shades.

GOOD CLEAN FUN

As with all the other categories of products I've discussed in this book, the hair products I recommend are those with the highest concentrations of natural ingredients and essential oils, and with the lowest amount of synthetic contents. This goes for everything from shampoo to hair coloring. I also implore you to use nonaerosol hair sprays, such as pumps and cans with air bladders, like AVEDA's Air-o-sol hair sprays. All aerosols release harmful propellants that have a cumulative, negative effect on the ozone layer and our air quality.

A small amount of preservatives and petrochemicals is necessary when we deal with products that are mostly natural; natural products would spoil otherwise, and the essential oil content necessary to fend off all the bacteria in the corner of the average bathtub would tend to irritate our skin. A low concentration of synthetic preservatives in AVEDA products ensures that they don't become inhabited by harmful bacteria, yeast, and fungi in your bathroom. Lots of the smaller companies, which sell natural shampoos and other cosmetics through health food stores, boast on their packaging that they use no preservatives. As a result, when we at AVEDA have tested

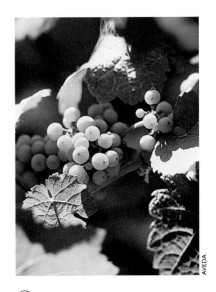

Grapes are another fruitful source of color that is gentle to you and your surroundings.

their products, we have always found them to be highly contaminated. In any case, the more natural the ingredients that go into our hair-care products, the better—for our hair, for the environment, and for the skin with which our hair products come into contact.

What's more, using shampoos, conditioners, and other hair products that contain essential oils allows us to have the additional benefits of aromatherapy, while also enjoying the stimulating or calming effects those essences have on our scalps and skin. There's also the wonderful effect plant-derived ingredients have on the hair and scalp. Hair gets cleaner, shines more, and generally looks healthier when it is cleaned, conditioned, and styled with natural products. Using natural products makes doing our hair a nurturing daily practice.

The first thing I do to my hair each day is something some people might think is the opposite of what should be done: I fill it with oil—pure jojoba oil with a few drops of essential oils that contain energizing properties. As I do my self–scalp massage, I'm also conditioning my hair the best possible way. Oil left on the hair through the morning exercise is a great way to restore moisture to our hair and protect it from the sun, wind, and free radicals all day long. A little bit of that oil will remain after the hair is washed and will act as a protective coat. Using a special, detoxifying shampoo once a week will remove any buildup of this oil.

On a daily basis, we should use shampoos made with pure plant essences, provitamin B5, and antioxidants like vitamin E. The shampooing experience should be enjoyed, slowly. Breathe in the fragrances of the essences, and feel their effects on the scalp and skin. Be conscious of how this feels and how it nurtures.

Shampooing should be followed with conditioning. In the shower, we use a conditioner that gets washed out, and this conditioner is really only

Massage an essential oil blend into any hair type to moisturize and protect.

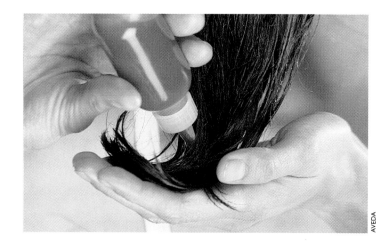

AVEDA

a small factor in how our hair winds up looking. That shower conditioner makes our hair more manageable and helps us to get a comb though it. In fact, you should comb the conditioner through your hair before rinsing it out. This smoothes the cuticle of the hair shaft down into its proper position. After you've massaged and combed the conditioner in, then rinse it out with cool, rather than hot, water, to keep the cuticle from rising again.

Now we come to the leave-in conditioners, fixatives, and pomades that we put in after we shower and that will have a greater effect on the way our hair performs. Of course, the texture of our hair has a lot to do with what it will do as we style it as well. Whether our hair is oily or dry, curly or straight, thick or thin, will determine what our best options for leave-in styling are. We can tailor our hair care and styling to suit our hair type.

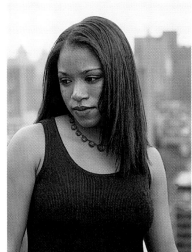

*T*hick, *highly textured hair benefits from a gentle shampoo and deep conditioner.*

CURLY, STRAIGHT, THICK, COARSE . . .

There are many variables that make one head of hair unique from another. There's the condition of the scalp—oily, dry, or normal. There's the thickness and actual density and diameter of each piece of hair. Finally, there's the texture, which determines how much straightness or wave the hair has to it.

The condition of the hair is another factor. Hair that is damaged and has its cuticles sticking up tends to look dull. The reason for this is that the broken up, haphazardly situated cuticles reflect light in many random directions. When the hair cuticle lies down smoothly, light is reflected uniformly and hair looks shinier. When the light does not scatter, we get healthy-looking hair. Proper conditioning, in and out of the shower, is key to promoting shiny hair. Combing those conditioners through in a downward motion to smooth down the cuticles is another key.

Today there are so many hair cleaning and styling products available that selecting one can be a confusing task. Look for natural plant essences in the ingredients, for they will give your hair and spirit a boost. From there, further define your goal for cleaning and setting. Shampoos go from mild to strong in their cleansing activity. Conditioners can be light or heavy, containing oil or not. Choose the ones you use based on your hair type. Hairstyling products are either oil-based or water-based, and they are designed to either increase or decrease hair tensile strength. Hair oils, creams, sticks, pomades, and waxes are meant to decrease volume and smooth hair. Sprays, gels, and mousses are meant to increase volume or texturize it.

*T*hick, medium-textured hair responds
well to water- or oil-based styling products. Take your pick!

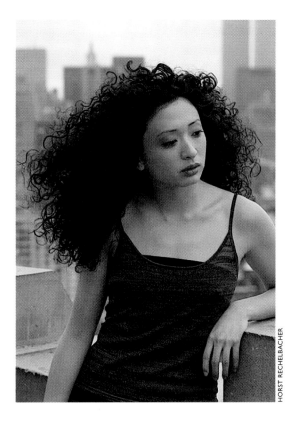

HORST RECHELBACHER

Hair type determines which type of styling product is preferable for
you. Here's a guide to hair types and the types of products that work best
for them:

Thin/Fine Hair

People with fine or thin hair should be careful not to overcondition their
hair. They should use a shampoo that's highly cleansing and a conditioner
that's light. A leave-in conditioner might be too much and have a tendency
to weigh down this type of hair. To add shine to thin/fine hair, use a water-
based or low-alcohol styling gel or a volumizing spray. Alcohol has been
given a bad name by some companies in the industry, but it can be useful in
adding volume to thin hair.

Thick, Medium Texture

People with thick, medium-textured hair can use a shampoo with more
active cleansing properties and a medium-weight conditioner. They can use
leave-in conditioners and styling products that are either water- or oil-
based. Lots of choices here.

Coarse, Highly Textured Hair That's Fine, Including African-Type Hair

Hair that's curly and coarse but fine is prone to damage. This type of hair requires a very gentle shampoo and a heavy conditioner. Styling products should be oil-based, and geared toward decreasing volume. You can also condition your hair by massaging some jojoba oil mixed with essential oils into your scalp before you shower. Comb the oil through so that the cuticle of the hair will lie down.

Coarse, Highly Textured Hair That's Thick

Hair that's curly and coarse but thick will require deep conditioning. The conditioner, as well as the styling products, should be oil-based. But because this hair doesn't damage easily, it can take a highly active shampoo.

DETOXIFY

All types of hair should be cleaned extrathoroughly with a detoxifying shampoo now and then. If you live in a city and are exposed there to a high level of pollutants, you might want to do this at least once a week. The same goes for those of you who daily style your hair with lots of product—or if you

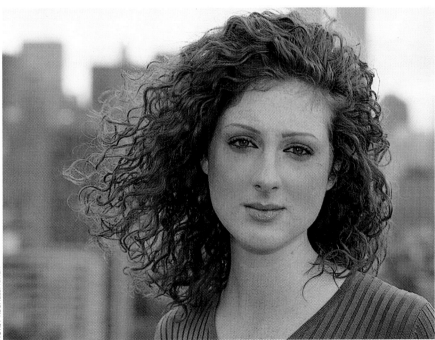

HORST RECHELBACHER

Give city hair a boost with a detoxifying shampoo once a week.

POTENTIALLY HARMFUL INGREDIENTS NOT USED BY AVEDA

PRODUCTS IN WHICH THESE INGREDIENTS ARE OFTEN INCLUDED	CTFA NAME	REASONS
Petrochemical nail polish	4-tert-Butyl Phenol, Formaldehyde Resin, Dibutyl Phthalate	Additives used in nail polish. Can cause skin depigmentation and allergic contact dermatitis.
Plant extracts	Benzene, Toluene, Xylene	Solvents derived from petrochemical fractionation.
Soap preservative	Butylated hydroxyanisole (BHA), Butylated Hydroxytoluene (BHT)	Petrochemical with antioxidant properties. Shown to impair blood clotting. Carcinogenic in animals. Associated with allergies in humans.
Shampoos and kitchen detergents	C_9 to C_{60} Pareth Surfactants	Synthetic alcohols reacted with ethylene oxide. Used as detergents for personal and household care. Aggressive surfactants may cause skin irritation.
Antiseptic cleansers	Hexachlorophene	Synthetic topical antiseptic with potential neurotoxicity in humans. FDA now regulates (bans) use.
Mousses and hairsprays	Isobutane, Isopentane	Aerosol propellants derived from petrochemical refineries. Respiratory and inhalation concerns.
Pomade	Isoparaffin, Paraffin, C_9 to C_{60} Alcohol	Long-chain fatty waxes derived from petrochemical refineries. Very poor biodegradation, pollution concerns.
Hair colors	Isopropyl Alcohol, Nonoxynol, Octoxynol	Petrochemical solvent made from propylene hydration. Synthetic surfactants. Petrochemical reacted with ethylene oxide.
Synthetic fragrances	Musk Xylene, Musk Tibetine, Musk Moskene	Synthetic nitro musk used as a fragrance fixative in soap and detergents. Health concerns include photoallergy and allergic contact dermatitis.
Sunscreens	Para-aminobenzoic Acid (PABA)	Sunscreens. Shown to be photoallergens.
All cosmetics for skin care and hair care	Propylene Glycol, Butylene Glycol	Petrochemical solvents made from propylene hydration. Employed as "industrial antifreeze." May cause contact urticaria and systemic contact dermatitis, and produce eczematous skin reactions.
Shampoos	Sodium C_{14} to C_{16} Olefin Sulfonate	High-foam irritating surfactant used in shampoos and cleansers. Derived from sulfonation of petrochemicals.
Hair conditioners	Tallow Trimonium Chloride, Hydrogenated Ditallowamine, Acetylated Hydrogenerated Tallow Glyceride	Derivatives of animal tallow (fat). Used in shampoos, conditioners, and fabric softeners.
Soaps, surfactants, shampoos	Triethanolamine, Diethanolamine	Made from ethylene oxide. Carcinogenic concerns associated with nitrosamine formation. Can cause allergic contact dermatitis.

frequently swim in chlorinated pools. A good detoxifying shampoo, which will contain highly active cleansers, can remove pollutants, oil buildup, and shampoo residue. But this sort of shampoo should probably not be used more than once a week, as it can be very active on the hair and the scalp. If you use a detoxifying shampoo too often, you'll be overcleaning your hair with a very strong cleanser that lacks conditioners. As a result, your hair can lose its pliability and shine, and ultimately break.

HAIR REPAIR

It should be noted that there is hope for restoring health to even the most damaged hair. Hair can take a lot of abuse before it is beyond repair. Our hair is born with a certain degree of resistance to damage. However, certain chemical treatments, such as overbleaching, perming and double-process coloring, will do irreparable harm. That is why it is so important to go to stylists who know what they are doing, who use products that are the least harmful to the hair and skin.

COLOR ME NATURAL

Hair color need not be completely artificial. We all know about tinting the hair with hennas, natural vegetable hair colorants that have been around since the time of the ancient Egyptians. These organic substances can be combined with a small amount of certain synthetics to create a more potent hair color that's more natural and less damaging to the hair, skin, and the air we breathe than most hair-color products used today.

AVEDA has been very successful in finding colors right in the ground, in the rain forest. We use these colors, from blue and black malva flowers, cherry bark, walnut shell oil, grapes, beets, and other plant life, in our semipermanent hair coloring as well as in shampoos and conditioners that are geared toward maintaining color. These natural sources deposit color into the hair without damaging it, and without threatening the environment.

Standard, highly synthetic hair coloring can be very harmful. Some of these products have lead bases. The FDA recently performed a thorough investigation into the ingredients in traditional hair colors. They found some of these hair colors contain several chemicals that are known carcinogens. Since then, many of the companies that make those products have continued to use these harmful substances but just renamed the chemicals

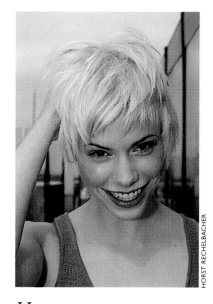

*H*air color can now be changed with 97 percent nonsynthetic materials; vegetable- and mineral-based dyes and essential oils change color and condition as well.

to disguise them. The FDA spent a fortune on this investigation and is not apt to do so again any time soon to ensure those items are removed. So, you should be very careful when selecting your hair-color products. Avoid using ones that contain ingredients from the table on page 136.

The safest hair colors are the lighter shades, because they are less concentrated. Darker colors have more toxins and synthetic chemical dyes. Even with hair colors that have more natural ingredients, the lighter colors are less harmful. AVEDA makes hair colors that are composed of 97 percent nonsynthetic materials, and that have had no carcinogenic effects. They contain vegetable- and mineral-based dyes and essential oils. Because they're made with essential oils, they smell much nicer than those other hair colors. And, in fact, the vegetable dyes are good for the hair. They coat the hair, and the essential oils nourish it. To choose what's right for you in terms of hair color, you need to consult with people who are very knowledgeable about these types of products. You might say this would be a hair "coach," much like the coaches I've recommended you consult for your other nurturing daily habits.

STYLE COUNCIL

Our hair coaches should also be people whom you can expect to guide you into styles that make you feel good about yourself, and make you feel like *yourself*. Hairstylists who don't listen to what you want to have done or what you hope to achieve with your hair don't deserve your patronage. If you leave someone's chair with the hair that he or she wanted to give you but not the hair that you wanted, you've gone to the wrong place. It doesn't matter how good other people say you look.

I don't recommend going to chain salons or salons where the owner is often absent. There tends to be a higher degree of professionalism and pride in a shop where the owner is present. In those salons, stylists are more likely to be knowledgeable about the limitations of certain hair types, as well as styling techniques and chemical processes. Choose a salon where the clients and the hairstylists appear to share your aesthetic sensibilities, but where there's also a sense of fashion-forwardness. You want stylists who can help you look current, if that's what you want.

Our coaches in all areas of our lives should be people who are interested in using their greater knowledge to help us on the journey back to ourselves—to our best selves. Look for this caring and concern before you settle on a hairstylist.

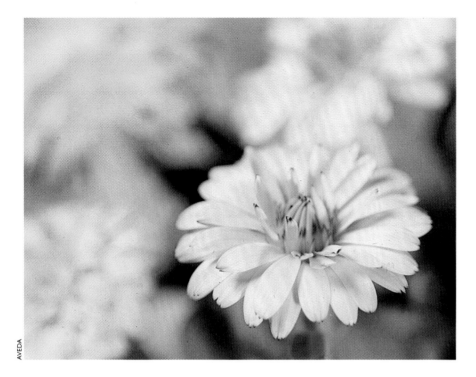

AVEDA

Calendula is an orange-yellow flower that brightens blond highlights and bathes hair and scalp with protective beta-carotene.

I also feel it is important to find a hairstylist who has the patience and vision to help you articulate what you want your hair to look like. I learned long ago that every client knows exactly what he or she wants once they get it, but that most have a hard time expressing it before they get into the chair. When I was cutting hair, I would always have clients show me pictures in magazines and hairstyling books I provided and talk to me about their lifestyle. If they were considering a change in length or texture, I would ask them about their mental associations with short and long styles, curly and straight textures. I found that it was important to find out *exactly* how short was short in their minds when they were looking to lose some length, or I'd wind up with angry clients with crew cuts when they wanted bobs.

Over the years, I became aware that clients and hairdressers were exposed on a daily basis to substances that could be harmful to them. Many hairdressers develop chronic diseases of the lungs, liver, kidneys, and skin from overexposure to toxic chemicals. My own daughter got blood poisoning from the formulas for a chemical wave when she worked at a hair salon in Europe. These factors alerted me to the choices a manufacturer has in formulating healthful or harmful hair products. I was inspired to use my knowledge of herbal medicine to broaden my scope and create hair products that would be good for the hair, the skin, the environment—and the hairstylist. AVEDA is the result.

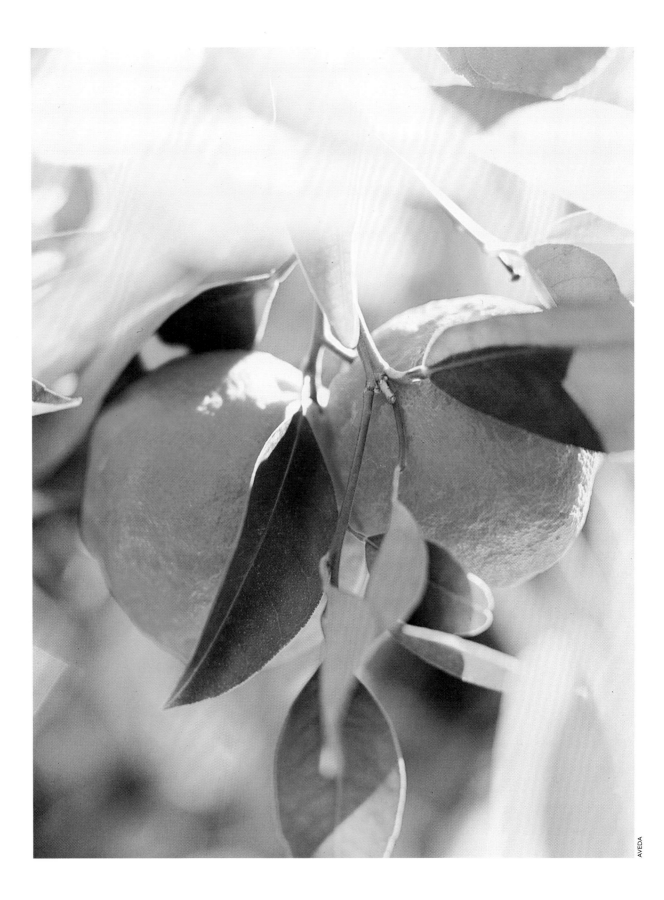

Midday Live

*Refocusing and Refreshing
Throughout the Day*

*Let us then be up and doing, and doing to the purpose; so by diligence
shall we do more with less perplexity.*

— BENJAMIN FRANKLIN

A WONDERFUL MORNING FILLED WITH HEALTHY NUR-
turing habits is a great way to start a day. But that alone is
no guarantee of momentum, of energy or spirit, for the rest
of the day. Just as breakfast provides a good starter meal but
certainly not enough food to satisfy or nourish us for a whole
twenty-four hours, our morning daily rituals need to be followed up later in
the day, with additional rejuvenating practices.

Once we've been at work for a while, or running our home—or even
enjoying a day of leisure—we reach a point at which we need to recharge
our batteries. We have drained ourselves of a lot of energy. We need to reenergize ourselves in some conscious way, through all our senses.

One way to reenergize is with a meal. We all know how to do that. Very
few people are not familiar with the concept of a lunch break. But it is not
just the body that needs to be rejuvenated. The mind and spirit require midday refortification, too. So, in the same way that you give your body a snack,
you can give your soul some morsels of restoration.

Most days, I take my practices from the morning and encapsulate them into smaller ones for the midmorning or the afternoon. When my attention and energy are lagging just before lunch, or later in the day, I incorporate one or more of the following:

- breathing exercises
- self-massage
- mirroring
- meditation
- motion
- aromatherapy

I might choose to participate in just one, a few, or all of the above, depending on the amount of time I have.

I try to consider my daytime rituals as I make my schedules. It's helpful to plan for these midday activities. I know that fatigue is not something we plan. But we all know our energy patterns fairly well. Most people lag in energy around 11 A.M. and again at 3 to 4 P.M. If we include our rituals in our scheduling, chances are we'll be more apt to stick to them and, as a result, be more healthful and productive throughout the day.

I learned the value of planning from my teacher, Swami Rama. He was the most amazing time manager. He was totally consistent. He took half-hour naps at the same time daily. It was understood among his disciples that after a meal, he was unavailable to us until he performed his afternoon rituals, including meditation and that little nap. We knew that at 4 P.M., he would be accessible to us again, and that if he didn't attend to his afternoon practices, he wouldn't be as helpful in teaching us later. We should all realize the benefits of restorative time well spent.

FOOD FOR THOUGHT

Admit it—you sometimes skip lunch. Or, you eat lunch standing, or working at your desk, barely able to taste your food. In American society, where many people view time as nothing but money, a lot of people don't realize the importance of making time for a real lunch hour—or even just a half hour.

This time is not just important for eating. It's important for taking a break, a real mental break, from your work. It is amazing how much more productive we can be after we've had a little respite and, hopefully, gotten away from our desks.

I have a hard-and-fast rule about lunch, which I enforce not only for myself, but for the employees of AVEDA: NO ONE EATS AT HIS OR HER DESK.

There are two reasons for this. The first is that it is important really to depart from the work environment, physically and mentally. At AVEDA's Minneapolis headquarters, there's a nice cafeteria that serves tasty organic food and even has a pool table. It's much more pleasant to eat there, or out in a park or restaurant, than in front of a computer and telephone.

The second reason is that when we eat at our desks, we bring the aromatics of food into our work environment, and they interfere with the aromatics we've set up to nurture our minds and bodies throughout the day. Our chairs and our cubicles absorb the smells of food. So when we're trying to rejuvenate ourselves later in the day with some wonderful essential oil, our olfactory systems may be overtaken by the smell of yesterday's tomato soup. How unpleasant and distracting! It's also unfair to the people who work nearby us who might not want to smell your lunch for days to come.

Another rule I have, which I can enforce only for myself, is that I don't work during lunch. Even if I am engaged in a business lunch, there is no wheeling and dealing during the eating part of the meal. We have to realize that our bodies and minds need to work together. If our bodies are eating, but our minds are doing business, we are completely out of sync. While I eat, I like to practice mindfulness and notice my food as I eat it. I'll participate in light, pleasant conversation as I eat. But I don't engage in really serious matters then. Before or after I've eaten, that's when I can conduct business.

I also recommend allotting part of your lunch period to some movement. Leave yourself ten or fifteen minutes to go for a walk, to get away and let your mind and body get revitalized. If you work at a company that has an on-site gymnasium, you might do some yoga or light aerobics for the first half of your lunch hour, and eat during the rest.

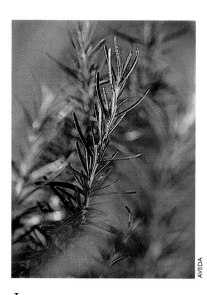

Instead of that candy bar you've come to depend upon, try refocusing afternoon energy by diffusing rosemary oil in your office.

AFTERNOON DELIGHT

When the 3 or 4 P.M. drop in blood sugar hits, what do you do? Do you run (or crawl) to the vending machine? Do you put your head down on the desk and hope nobody notices? While these options might have worked for you in the past, I've got some slightly healthier recommendations you might want to consider:

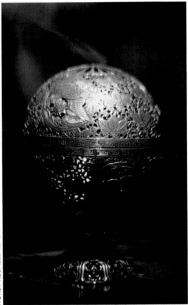

*T*ry *lighting cypress or cedar in a beautiful burner like this one. It's an aesthetic break that's invigorating to mind, body, and spirit.*

▶ Sniff some essential oils that you love in order to arouse your mind, which will in turn awaken your body.

▶ Do some breathing exercises.

▶ Remember that scalp massage your learned to give yourself in the morning? Or the all-over self-massage? Do an even shorter version at your desk, and you'll perk up in a much more balanced way than you would from the caffeine in a Diet Coke.

▶ While you might not be able to do the entire solar salutation yoga routine at your desk, executing just a few yoga postures, some with inversion, can get your blood moving again, while also revitalizing your mind and spirit.

▶ Take a ten-minute walk around the outside of your building to clear your mind and help your body to wake up.

▶ Once you've stimulated your mind and body a bit with some movement, massage or aromatherapy, meditate on your goals for the day so that you can stay connected with your intentions.

When you bring your new habits into your whole day, you create a continuity that supports your wellness, all around. Your mind, body, and spirit need conscious nurturing—not just sometimes, but morning, noon, and night, every day.

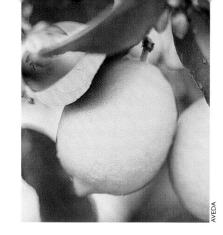

Nourished by Nature

Balance, Organics, Supplements

I follow nature as the surest guide, and resign myself with implicit obedience, to her sacred ordinances.

—CICERO

O F ALL THE HABITS WE CREATE IN DESIGNING A NEW set of nurturing practices, how we eat can have some of the most profound and noticeable effects on us. While all our positive habits contribute to an improved quality of life and appearance—from our self-massages to our exercise and natural skin care—eating right can most profoundly change how we think, feel, and look.

It is very easy to read how someone is eating from the shape of their body and from their complexion. When we change the way we eat, our appearance soon changes as well. If we improve our diet—eliminating the wrong fats and including the right ones, lowering intake of sodium, sugar, and artificial ingredients as much as possible, and balancing protein and carbohydrate—chances are we will trim down, firm up, and glow more.

There has been a shift in recent years toward somewhat healthier eating in Western cultures. Because our society places such an importance on thinness, many people have switched to low-fat and low-sugar diets. Our general awareness has increased regarding the ills of high cholesterol, and the key role vegetables play in fighting cancer. These are positive steps, for sure. But many of those who are cutting fat are increasing sodium intake through processed foods. They're also eating more vegetables, but more often than not, those vegetables are not organic; the insecticides, pesticides, artificial fertilizers, and poor soil they grew in have depleted their vitamin and mineral content. If not washed, they also can be covered with carcinogenic insecticides. Therefore, in the end, some of those vegetables that are being eaten to prevent cancer are actually capable of causing it.

THE ORGANIC IMPERATIVE

At various points throughout this book, you will notice that I have mentioned the importance of supporting organic farming. I can't stress this enough.

When we eat fruits and vegetables that are grown organically, we provide our bodies with food that hasn't been treated with pesticides, and that is much richer in vital nutrients. In short, the microcosm, the self, is nurtured by organic food.

The macrocosm, the planet, is nurtured by organics, too. We live in a closed system here on Earth. The pesticides that are sprayed on nonorganic foods make their way around the world and into our lives through not only the food we eat, but the water we drink and the air we breathe as well. So, even if we do make a point of buying and eating only organically as a world population, we will have to contend with the harmful effects of pesticides for years to come. These carcinogenic chemicals are airborne; they enter the water supply and are distributed around the world as the foods that bear them are exchanged among continents.

In situations where only nonorganic produce is available, I recommend washing it very thoroughly with soap and water. Peel those fruits and vegetables with particularly thin skins. But be aware that pesticides can't always be washed off or peeled away with the skin of a fruit or vegetable. Many of the newer chemicals being used are genetically engineered to make their way into the root systems of plants, and are coded to assimilate into the seeds. So they will find their way into every part of the fruits and vegetables you eat.

What's more, pesticides deplete the soil of its nutrients. The insects the pesticides are designed to kill are actually vital to soil and the plants that grow in it. Many of the nutrients in organic food are provided by the waste those insects produce. Once the soil is depleted of such nutrients, it dies and no longer provides life.

Regulations restricting the use of pesticides are flimsy. DDT, a pesticide that has been banned in the United States for decades, is actually in much of the food sold here. It's on our food because other countries use it on all sorts of crops, including coffee and tea, and the FDA doesn't monitor the pesticides used on food that is imported. DDT has a number of very harmful effects, and it is a very potent carcinogen that also reduces the sperm count in men and generally weakens the immune system of anyone who comes into contact with it. With our global economy, we are no longer free from harmful substances such as DDT unless every county bans them.

It is a wise activity to support organic farming; it does not use harmful chemicals and it replenishes the soil, making it rich in nutrients that are then absorbed by the fruits and vegetables grown on it. Organic farming doesn't harm the environment or the water supply, and the natural intelligence of the foods grown without added chemicals is left intact. Today, organic foods are slightly more expensive because demand for them is lower, and it costs farmers more to harvest them naturally than to harvest nonorganic crops. If more of us support organic farming, the costs of those foods will likely decrease. It is for our global benefit that we stand behind the production of organic foods with our choices and our dollars.

I have learned a lot about the ecological benefits of organics from a brilliant man named Teri Gips, one of the founders of the Alliance for Sustainability. I met him when he was a part-time professor at the University of Minnesota where I took some environmental ecology courses. He wrote a book called *The Dirty Dozen*, about the dangerous chemicals that are in food and that we should try to avoid. Through him I have learned a tremendous amount about the importance of corporate and social practices that support sustainability of natural resources. Citizens, manufacturers, and society as a whole can adopt behaviors and lifestyles that are less harmful to our world and that encourage the continued existence of the nature on which we rely. Supporting organic farming and eating only organic foods is a key part of the formula. It's a way for each one of us as individuals to become internal and external activists. Educating others takes our support a step further.

AMERICA'S MOST UNWANTED

In this chapter I've mentioned DDT, a pesticide banned in the United States, which inadvertently appears in much of our food anyway since it's not banned in many of the countries from which we import. There are many other pesticides, legal in the United States and elsewhere, that we can avoid when we eat organically. *The Catalogue of Healthy Food,* by John Tepper Marlin with Domenick M. Bertelli, mentions the following partial list:

▶ acephate—a carcinogen and mutagen commonly used on celery, legumes, and peppers that cannot be washed off

▶ alachlor—a carcinogen used widely on corn, peanuts, and soybeans in the United States

▶ aldicarb—a highly toxic insecticide used on potatoes, citrus fruits, and soybeans that cannot be washed off

▶ captan—a carcinogen and mutagen used as a fungicide on apples, cherries, grapes, peaches, and strawberries

▶ chlorothalonil—a carcinogen, mutagen, and catalyst for several chronic disease effects used as a fungicide on cantaloupes, cauliflower, celery, legumes, tomatoes, and watermelon

▶ ethylene bisdithiocarbamates (EBDCs)—a fungicide used on one-third of all U.S. fruits and vegetables

▶ lindane—a carcinogen and catalyst for chronic disease effects used on leafy vegetables; the same formula as used in Kwell, the remedy for head lice

▶ methyl parathion—a carcinogen, mutagen, and catalyst for chronic disease effects that is commonly used on cantaloupes and strawberries

▶ parathion—a carcinogen and mutagen used on broccoli, carrots, cherries, oranges, and peaches

▶ permethrin—a carcinogen used on sixty crops including corn, soybeans, and tomatoes

▶ phosmet—a carcinogen and mutagen used on apples, pears, and sweet potatoes

▶ trifluralin—a carcinogen and catalyst for chronic disease effects that is used on carrots and that cannot be washed off

In addition to avoiding pesticides, certified organic foods avoid the following other harmful additives:

▶ growth regulators such as the highly publicized Alar

▶ chemical fertilizers

- antibiotics fed to livestock to keep them bacteria-free (drawback: antibiotics become less effective in the humans who consume meat or dairy from these animals)

- salmonella, which grows more rampantly in chickens that are kept too close together, in unsanitary conditions, and/or are fed the parts of other dead chickens

- hormones such as Bovine Growth Hormone (BGH), designed to increase the milk output of cows, but which can create hormonal effects and allergies in the humans who drink that milk

- preservatives such as BHA and BHT

- artificial colors

- emulsifiers

- stabilizers

- flavor enhancers

- artificial sweeteners

- irradiation, which depletes some nutrients in food, creates carcinogens in some foods, and often leads to contamination accidents at irradiation plants

INTO THE MOUTHS OF BABES

The danger of pesticides is not limited to fresh foods. Pesticides and other harmful chemicals can be found in many packaged foods as well, which is why it is important to look for certified organics in *all* our foods.

As an example, Teri Gips of the Alliance for Sustainability has provided the following list of sixteen pesticides commonly found in baby food—three of which are probable carcinogens, five of which are possible carcinogens, eight of which are neurotoxins, five of which are endocrine disruptors, and five of which are categorized as "oral toxicity 1 chemicals," the most highly toxic designation there is:

- acephate
- amothoate
- azinphos methyl
- botran
- carbaryl
- chlorpyriphos
- DDE
- DDT
- dieldrin
- dimethoate
- endosulfan
- ethion
- iprodione
- methamidiphos
- methyl parathion
- permethrin
- thiabendazole

A DELICATE BALANCE

Once we make the switch to organics, we have other decisions to make about our eating habits.

▪ Do we want to maintain or lose weight and/or reshape our bodies?

▪ Do we want to try a vegetarian diet?

▪ What are the right ratios of carbohydrate to protein, and fat to fiber?

It is rare to meet someone these days who isn't interested in weight loss, or weight maintenance through diet. At the moment, doctors I know and respect recommend a diet that features a ration of at least 60 percent protein to 40 percent carbohydrate for natural optimal weight maintenance, as well as prevention of heart disease and cancer. If you're a nonvegetarian, look to low-fat animal protein sources, like fish and white-meat chicken, to get your protein. But don't eliminate all fat. These doctors also recommend that you include some essential fatty acids, like those found in fish and olive, hemp, or flax seed oil, in each meal. These acids help to lower triglycerides and increase levels of good cholesterol in the blood. Naturally, fruits and vegetables are also an important component of this recommended diet. In fact, the doctors suggest that cancer-preventing fruits and vegetables should constitute about one-third of all food we enjoy.

FOOD AS MEDICINE

Food is not only nourishment. It is also an important weapon against dis-ease and disease. Here are ten foods that are particularly powerful medicinal edibles—and you probably won't have to go much farther than your own refrigerator to find most of them:

Tomatoes

Sliced or pureed, in salads or sauces, tomatoes are one of the healthiest vegetables around. They're rich in *p*-coumaric acid and chlorogenic acid, which can hook on to nitrites in the foods we eat and spirit them out of the system before they team up with amines to form cancer-causing nitrosamines. Tomatoes are also abundant in the antioxidant lycopene, which is thought to protect against cancers of the colon and bladder. Good thing tomatoes happen to be one of the most popular vegetables around, as well.

EVIDENCE THAT IT WORKS

When researchers combined an experimental concoction of *p*-coumaric acid, chlorogenic acid, and amines, the production of nitrosamines fell by about 20 percent. A recent Italian study found that people who ate raw tomatoes at least seven times a week halved their risk of several cancers, compared to those who ate tomatoes no more than once a week.

WHAT ELSE IS GOOD

Watermelons, grapefruits, and carrots contain lycopene. *P*-coumaric and chlorogenic acids can be found in green peppers, strawberries, and carrots.

ADDITIONAL BENEFITS

Tomatoes are good sources of vitamin C, beta-carotene, and potassium, which can help protect against heart disease.

Garlic

The chemicals called allium compounds, which give garlic and onions their distinctive tang, boost levels of naturally occurring enzymes that detoxify potential carcinogens. Allium compounds may also stimulate cancer-fighting immune cells.

EVIDENCE THAT IT WORKS

In China's Shandong Province, epidemiologists have found that people who consume large amounts of garlic and onions cut their risk of stomach cancer by as much as 40 percent. Closer to home, a study of more than 41,000 women in Iowa showed that those who added garlic to the menu at least once a week reduced their risk of colon cancer by 35 percent. Other studies have shown that garlic can inhibit the growth of tumors of the esophagus, rectum, and skin.

WHAT ELSE IS GOOD

Scallions and chives.

ADDITIONAL BENEFITS

Several ingredients in garlic appear to reduce the "stickiness" of blood platelets, preventing the kinds of clots that can lead to heart attacks. By preventing platelets from sticking to artery walls, garlic may also reduce the risk of hardening of the arteries.

In a study review by researchers at New York Medical College in Valhalla, people who ate the equivalent of one clove of garlic a day saw their cholesterol levels drop about 9 percent. That translates to an almost 20 percent reduction in heart disease risk.

Soybeans

Poor soybeans. Ground into flour or shaped into cubes of tofu, they don't play a big part in the American diet. But that may change. Scientists have discovered that soy is rich in a substance called genistein, which protects against cancer in several ways.

EVIDENCE THAT IT WORKS

Cancer cells in the breast and ovary are stimulated by estrogen, and genistein, an estrogen look-alike, can step in instead, plugging up receptors for the hormone. Genistein may also prevent small blood vessels from forming around cancer cells, cutting off oxygen and nutrients. A 1994 study found that a diet rich in soy protein lengthens the menstrual cycle in women by roughly a day and a half, reducing exposure to estrogen. That could explain why Japanese women have one-fourth the rate of breast cancer as Americans.

WHAT ELSE IS GOOD

Along with tofu, soy flour, soy milk, and especially miso, genistein shows up in peanuts, mung beans, and alfalfa sprouts.

ADDITIONAL BENEFITS

Low in sodium and cholesterol-free, soybeans are a terrific source of protein.

Grapes

Grapes are one of the oldest cultivated fruits, dating all the way back to Neolithic times. Today, scientists are discovering new reasons to savor the fruit of the vine. Grapes are loaded with ellagic acid, which blocks the body's production of enzymes that cancer cells need to grow.

EVIDENCE THAT IT WORKS

In mice, an extract of Concord grapes has been shown to be as effective as the cancer drug methotrexate in slowing tumor growth.

WHAT ELSE IS GOOD

Apples, strawberries, and raspberries.

ADDITIONAL BENEFITS

Apples may get top billing in folklore, but researchers say grapes are packed with plenty of healthful chemicals beside ellagic acid, such as phenols, antioxidants that may prevent blood clots. Red grape skins also contain resveratrol, a natural fungicide that slows the buildup of "bad" LDL cholesterol.

Oranges and Lemons

Scientists have identified a substance plentiful in oranges, lemons, and limes called limonene, which boosts levels of naturally occurring enzymes thought to break down carcinogens and stimulate cancer-killing immune cells. Citrus fruits also contain glucarase, which inactivates carcinogens and speeds them out of the body.

EVIDENCE THAT IT WORKS

Pure limonene has been shown to reduce and prevent tumors in mice. Orange juice may work almost as well. When mice exposed to a potent carcinogen lapped up the juice—the equivalent for you of about a gallon a day—they developed 40 percent fewer early signs of cancer than mice on a juiceless diet.

WHAT ELSE IS GOOD

Limonene is also plentiful in cardamom, celery, and the seeds of caraway and fennel.

ADDITIONAL BENEFITS

High in vitamin C, oranges, lemons, and other citrus fruits may boost fertility and encourage the production of healthy sperm in men. Studies at the University of California at Berkeley have found that vitamin C protects sperm from damage by oxidation.

Licorice Root

The word *licorice* originally comes from the Greek, meaning "sweet root." In fact, the principal ingredient in licorice, called glycyrrhizin, is fifty times sweeter than table sugar. It may also be a potent defense against cancer.

EVIDENCE THAT IT WORKS

Glycyrrhizin prevents testosterone from changing into a form that has been shown to trigger prostate cancer. Glycyrrhizin also seems to protect DNA from damage caused by carcinogens and may even boost cancer-killing immune cells. Mice who lapped up water laced with glycyrrhizin and were then exposed to a strong carcinogen were far less likely to develop tumors than mice given plain water. The tumors that did appear were smaller and appeared significantly later.

WHAT ELSE IS GOOD

European licorice still contains the real thing, but in the United States most licorice twists are flavored with anise, not licorice. Don't overindulge. Dangerously high blood pressure and other problems have been seen in people who gobble thirty-five to forty bite-sized licorice candies daily for weeks or months on end.

ADDITIONAL BENEFITS

Licorice guards the stomach wall against ulcers by stimulating the production of a protective lining of mucus.

Green Tea

" 'Take some more tea,' the March Hare said to Alice, very earnestly," in Lewis Carroll's classic tale. It may be good advice. Tea leaves are laced with substances called polyphenols—antioxidants that can prevent the kind of damage to DNA that leads to cancer. When cancer cells do form, one group of polyphenols, called catechins, seem to prevent them from multiplying. Catechins may also trap carcinogens and speed them out of the body.

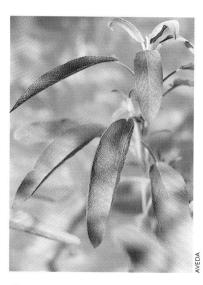

Sage is thought by Native American tribes to rid a place of negative spirits. Use it to cleanse the air and energize your thoughts.

EVIDENCE THAT IT WORKS

Mice given green tea in their drinking water developed half the expected number of lung tumors when exposed to a carcinogen in tobacco smoke. Results from human studies have been less clear. Still, researchers are intrigued by studies like one in Shanghai, in which one group of tea drinkers cut their risk of cancer of the esophagus by more than half compared to non–tea drinkers.

WHAT ELSE IS GOOD

Green or black—but not herbal—tea. Let your cup cool a bit, though. One study showed an increased risk of esophageal cancer among tea drinkers, and most scientists put the blame on a habit of taking the beverage boiling hot.

Artichokes

The thistle known as an artichoke has been savored since the Middle Ages in Italy. Full of fiber, artichokes can help speed toxins or potential carcinogens out of the digestive system. Even more important, artichokes are one of the best sources of folic acid, which could help ward off cervical cancer.

EVIDENCE THAT IT WORKS

Low levels of folic acid appear to make cells of the cervix more vulnerable to human papilloma virus infection, which is thought to play a role in cervical cancer, according to researchers at the University of Alabama at Birmingham. Folic acid deficiency has also been associated with higher rates of dysplasia, a condition of abnormal cells in the cervix believed to be one of the early signs of trouble. Researchers at the University of Chicago Medical Center have found evidence that low levels of folic acid also increase the risk of colon cancer.

WHAT ELSE IS GOOD

Asparagus, beets, yeast breads, and liver are all rich in folic acid.

ADDITIONAL BENEFITS

Folic acid is also important for pregnant women, since researchers are convinced that adequate folic acid helps prevent neural-tube defects.

Artichokes may also help lower cholesterol. An anticholesterol drug was originally developed from a compound in artichokes called cynarin.

Hot Peppers

In salsas and sauces, stir-fries and spicy drinks, chile peppers are more popular than ever. Now researchers suspect that the hot stuff in peppers, called capsaicin, may also extinguish carcinogens before they cause trouble. A potent antioxidant, capsaicin prevents the deadly union of nitrites and amines that forms nitrosamines.

EVIDENCE THAT IT WORKS

When researchers mixed pure capsaicin into a witches' brew of nitrosamines, the carcinogenic substances were almost completely neutralized. Capsaicin may also keep carcinogens found in cigarette smoke from locking onto DNA, possibly preventing the genetic damage that can lead to lung and other cancers.

WHAT ELSE IS GOOD

The hotter the pepper, the more capsaicin it contains. Jalapeños are better than canned green chiles; fiery Thai peppers are better still.

ADDITIONAL BENEFITS

German researchers have found that by stimulating the flow of digestive juices, capsaicin seems to shield the stomach lining against damage from acids and alcohol. There's also good evidence that capsaicin can lower blood pressure. Add to that the fact that chiles are loaded with vitamins A and C, and you've got plenty of reason to turn up the heat.

Broccoli and Cabbage

"The cabbage surpasses all other vegetables," wrote the Roman poet Cato. Throw in cabbage's cruciferous cousins—including broccoli, kale, brussels sprouts, and cauliflower—and he just might be right. Crucifers contain a treasure trove of cancer-fighting substances. Brassinin and sulforaphane, for instance, boost the body's production of the enzymes that defuse potential carcinogens and then flush them out of the system. Substances called indoles affect the metabolism of estrogen, prompting the body to make benign forms of the hormone that don't promote breast cancer.

EVIDENCE THAT IT WORKS

University of Minnesota researcher Lee Wattenberg has shown that mice exposed to a strong carcinogen and then fed meals rich in broccoli or cabbage (the equivalent of your eating three-fourths of a pound a day) are half as likely to develop cancer as mice who've never munched a broccoli floret or crunched a cabbage leaf. In a 1991 study, twelve volunteers downed an indole-heavy vegetable extract every day for a week. Tests at week's end showed a 50 percent increase in blood levels of "good" estrogen.

Broccoli and other crucifers are especially rich in numerous antioxidants, including beta-carotene and vitamin C, which are believed to protect DNA from the kind of damage that can turn healthy cells cancerous.

WHAT ELSE IS GOOD

Brussels sprouts, cauliflower, bok choy, kale, mustard greens, radishes.

ADDITIONAL BENEFITS

Cruciferous vegetables are good sources of fiber, which can help reduce blood pressure and lower "bad" LDL cholesterol levels.

In order to lose weight, it is no secret that we must decrease our calorie intake and increase our calorie burning. We must reach a delicate balance of diet and exercise to maintain a metabolism that has enough fire to keep us burning energy. If we cut our calories too much, we risk slowing down our metabolism, which will counteract our weight-loss goals. Weight loss should be a slow, gentle process, in which we still allow ourselves plenty of the foods we like. Getting thin can make us feel very good about ourselves, but it's not so important that we should risk our health for it. In addition, weight that comes off more slowly and naturally tends to stay off. There's no rush.

Before beginning a weight-loss-oriented diet, we should think about our eating habits and why we eat. Many of us who overeat are likely to do so as a reaction to stress, loneliness, depression, anger, or boredom. In a daily mirroring session, be honest with yourself about why you might overeat. Being conscious and mindful of your eating attitudes and habits is a positive step toward making changes. If you are eating for reasons other than hunger, you can work to identify them and address unmet needs in another, more healthy way.

Consider how many times you eat a day. Most of us were raised with the idea of eating three square meals a day. Dr. Barry Sears, creator of the Zone Diet and author of books about it, has found that it is better to eat five smaller meals a day, plus two snacks when we want them. Our digestive systems are designed to process small amounts of food at a time. Our blood sugar levels remain stable, and we function more steadily when we do this sort of "grazing."

When we do eat, we should do it mindfully. That means paying attention to our eating and making it a nurturing ritual. Try lighting a candle while you eat or playing your favorite soothing music, or both! Make eating a sensual experience by not reading or watching television or doing anything else while you eat other than noticing how your food feels and tastes in your mouth. Observe yourself with regard to food. This subtle consciousness will most likely lead you to a new understanding and appreciation of food's place in your life. This, in turn, can lead you to take action toward new habits.

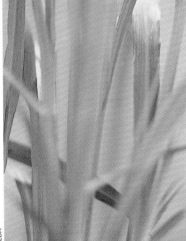

AVEDA

Lemongrass, a natural appetite suppressant

THE BEST DEFENSE

Our culture is obsessed with food—*bad* food. Magazines are filled with oddly juxtaposed ads for rich foods and articles about health and weight loss. Fast-food chains keep growing and expanding their reach to even the most remote corners all over the globe. No wonder we sometimes find it's hard to have a rational attitude toward food. A positive way to think about it involves our looking at it at its most basic: Food is fuel. The quality of the fuel we put in our bodies will affect the way our bodies run.

That means we should eat plenty of foods that energize the body. Organic foods provide more energy than nonorganic. When shopping in the supermarket, one helpful tip is to try to pick up a rainbow of color in your fruits and vegetables. This means you'll be picking up an array of vitamins and nutrients, which work together to boost energy. We need a good amount of protein in our diets—60 percent or more—balanced with some carbohydrate, fat, and fiber to keep energy up. We should eat a variety of foods to ensure a good balance of vitamins and minerals. Another important factor to consider is our elemental makeups, or Ayurvedic doshas, and the types of food that are specifically recommended for each. Refer to Chapter 3 to figure out your dominant doshas, and the foods that will work best with your constitution to give you the greatest energy.

No matter what your dosha, ginseng is great natural energy booster to add to your diet. So is spirulina, an algae with 65 percent protein that's especially useful in vegetarian diets. Herbs like cayenne and mustard, which are thermagenic, or create heat for energy, also have been used for ages by many cultures as energy herbs.

Including raw foods in our diet also increases energy and helps us digest all our other food. Raw foods possess enzymes that give the body the means for smooth digestion. Having something raw with each meal aids the flow of energy through the body because it facilitates our digestion and elimination processes.

SCENTS THAT SATISFY

Many of us feel hungry and look to food for nurturance when we experience loneliness, sadness, boredom, or other stressful emotions. We can satisfy this false sense of appetite with plant-based aromas. Which aromas will work the best? The ones you love, which you associate with feeling nurtured. However, some essential oils have appetite-suppressing qualities by nature. Among them are

▸ tangerine

▸ lemongrass

▸ clove in cinnamon

▸ citrus oils

▸ rose

▸ jasmine

▸ peppermint

▸ vanilla

▸ orange

SUPPLEMENTAL INCOME

Vegetarians, or those considering vegetarianism, should note that this mode of eating poses a challenge. If you are among the many who choose vegetarianism, you should be aware that this type of diet does make it more difficult to get all the protein you need. Whereas the typical American diet is filled with too much protein, usually from animal sources, the vegetarian diet has few sources of protein. If you go the vegetarian route, be sure to eat plenty of soy, beans, and legumes.

Even those of us who maintain perfectly balanced diets rich in organic foods might have trouble getting all the vitamins and minerals we need. To ensure our natural reserves it is smart to take herb and vitamin supplements, plenty of which should be antioxidants. Here are some you might consider adding to your medicine chest as regulars:

▸ The antioxidants A, C, and E fight free radicals from the inside. Wearing a makeup foundation with antioxidants is just not enough—free radicals can still make their way onto and into your body. We have to guard ourselves inside and out. But be careful not to overdose, particularly on vitamin A. Talk to the people behind the counter when you're purchasing vitamins for guidance about dosages.

▸ The B vitamins are good sources of energy and excellent for brain function.

▸ Saint-John's-wort is an antidepressant.

▸ Zinc boosts the immune system and helps heal prostate problems in men.

▸ Phytoestrogenic herbs, taken in capsules, tinctures, or teas, are helpful in quelling the effects of premenstrual syndrome (PMS) from which women can suffer. Among those herbs are wild yam, dong quai, and licorice root.

▸ Calming herbs like kava kava root and Siberian ginseng can heal us when we're stressed out.

▸ Valerian root, kava kava, chamomile, or California poppy will help combat insomnia.

▸ Green tea, as well as herbs such as peppermint, cardamom, lemongrass, and sage, peps us up. You can take these herbs as teas, tinctures, or in capsule form.

In the end you should try to remember that eating should be a pleasurable experience. When you make a concerted effort to prepare and eat a healthy, fresh, appealing variety of foods, you'll find it much easier to accomplish your eating plan. Do it to be happy and healthy.

REAL-LIFE WAYS TO EAT BETTER

Following are some tips regarding changing our eating habits so that eating becomes a practice that truly nurtures our mind, body, and spirit:

- Focus on less calories and fat, more exercise.

- Buy organic foods whenever possible.

- Drink eight to ten glasses of water daily. Two of these glasses should be consumed thirty minutes before meals to reduce appetite. Try squeezing lemon into your water to add flavor.

- Eat slowly and chew food well. A meal or snack should take twenty to thirty minutes to eat. Wait ten to fifteen minutes before taking a second helping.

- Limit treats and refined foods, minimize salt intake, reduce or avoid alcohol and caffeine, and avoid sodas and chemical foods.

- Become a label reader and use only low-fat or nonfat milk products.

- Eat a variety of foods.

- Learn how to use spices creatively and discover that flavor isn't synonymous with fat.

- Learn how to enjoy your food. Don't eat finger foods by the handful—eat them piece by piece to savor the flavor and the sensual experience of eating.

- Don't eat while standing or cooking.

- Eat all meals and snacks as scheduled. Don't skip meals or save up for one big meal.

- Treat yourself to a big (but healthy) breakfast. You have an entire day to burn off the calories.

- At restaurants, avoid buttered or oily foods or ask that foods be prepared accordingly.

- If you blow it, go right back on the plan. Do not make it an excuse for failure.

- Allow yourself to really enjoy the plan's scheduled snacks.

- Don't eat in front of the television or while reading.

- Take your own fat-free snack to the movie theater, or contribute a low-fat dish at a party.

- Don't be tempted to load your grocery cart with fat-free substitutes. Sometimes nutrients are lost with the fat. Remember, it is always best to choose naturally low-fat whole foods.

- Keep a food diary. If you notice problem foods that increase your appetite, avoid them. For example, you may find when you eat something sweet, or consume a specific grain or a particular kind of food, you actually become more hungry.

- Find low-fat recipes and start experimenting.

- Keep organic fresh fruits and vegetables in the house as snacks.

- Make lunch and take it with you to work along with fruits and/or vegetables as snacks so you can avoid the vending machine.

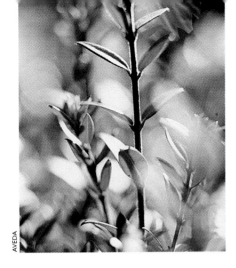

Herbal Renewal

What Pure Aromatherapy Really Is

Perfumes are the feelings of flowers.

—Heinrich Heine

OUR SENSE OF SMELL OFFERS US MUCH MORE THAN just the ability to stop and smell the roses. Our noses are gateways to our brains, and the natural fragrances we choose to breathe in work like intricate data with their ability to condition and program our minds. How our brains process that data depends partly on what they already know. There are scents that our experience has told us are positive and nurturing—like the smell of fresh-baked bread, or fresh-cut roses. As soon as we smell those things again, we are filled with the same warm, fuzzy feelings we had the first time we encountered them. There are also scents that we've learned to view as warning signs of unpleasantness—like the smell of spoiled milk, fire, or the smell of the antiseptic in the dentist's office. When we are exposed to those smells, our minds experience the same fear, anxiety, and pain we felt the first time we came upon them. No other physical clues beyond smell are needed for our minds to send out the stress-reaction impulses. Automatically, pheromones and endorphins bring this motivating information to the rest of our bodies. This is what is known in aromatherapy as *olfactory memory response*.

Natural scents also carry an inherent code that affects the mind and body independently of what the brain associates with it. For example, energizing essential oils—like rosemary, eucalyptus, and peppermint—awaken the senses whether or not the person breathing them in has had any prior exposure to them. Essences like vanilla, jasmine, and chamomile will calm regardless of the memory's associations with their scents. Certain plant properties carried in the gaseous molecules that are transmitted from them to us in the form of a smell affect our bodies' chemistry in a subtle, but powerful, manner.

THE REAL ROSE — TRUE PLANT AND FLOWER ESSENCES

There is a huge difference between natural fragrances and chemical mimics that we humans have made. Natural plant and flower essences are highly preferable to petrochemical compounds that are formulated to smell like the real thing. Our noses may not be able to immediately identify the real essence from its synthetic copy, but our brains can—and so can every cell in our bodies. Real plants and flowers and their essences carry information that the brain can understand. The brain's own yin (calming) and yang (stimulating) energies can be balanced by the yin and yang energies in plants and flowers. When we are in an extreme emotional state, we can use natural essences with opposite properties to calm or energize us as needed. It's the intricate data carried by the natural plant essences that tell our brains how to react, whether we've trained them to have certain responses to scents or not. The message of an essence is conveyed to the brain through the olfactory system, stimulating a reaction in the sympathetic and parasympathetic nervous systems that results in a corresponding psychological reaction.

While the fake fragrances can fool our noses for a brief while, they won't have a long-term effect on our state of being or on our behavior. Besides, the petrochemical compounds put stress on our noses and our brains, because they are synthetics that our body must work hard to rid itself of.

In order to have a better understanding of why it's so important to use products that contain real plant essences, it will be helpful first to

FOLLOW YOUR NOSE

What is the right oil or combination of oils to use as a deodorant? The answer is simple: those oils that smell good to you. I use jasmine, rose, neroli, orange, lemon, lemongrass, frankincense (or olibanum), peppermint, and lavender green because I love them.

There are some oils that are thought to be particularly pleasant and that have a way of upstaging life's less pleasant smells. Among them are

- bergamot
- caraway seed
- cassia
- chamomile
- citronella
- clary sage
- cypress
- eucalyptus
- fir
- jasmine
- laurel leaf
- lemongrass
- myrtle
- neroli
- orange
- palmarosa
- peppermint
- pine
- rose
- sage
- spearmint
- star anise
- tea tree
- thyme

understand exactly what those essences are. While lovely and very Edenlike, it would be incredibly expensive and nearly impossible to surround ourselves with fresh plants and flowers all the time, and to have their blooms added to everything we put on our skin and into our bodies. But there are ways to take the life energy and other properties of those plants and flowers and keep this energy and these properties alive for use in various substances. These processes are distillation and extraction. The prana, chi, ki, or life force, of fresh plants and flowers is distilled or extracted into what are called essential oils. But in a way, this is a misnomer, since there is no oil in most essential oils. (So you needn't worry about their leaving oil stains on fabrics.) To capture this essential oil from plants and flowers, we press and distill them in water while they are in full bloom, extracting the live information they contain and preserving it in liquid form. Although the original flower soon dies, its biological information stays alive in the form of an essence, as long as the essence is kept fresh. Light and heat can weaken or spoil essential oils by interfering with their chemical structures. That is why it is important to keep many essential oils in a cool, dark place. Different approaches are required to draw the essences from different plants and flowers because of their molecular structures. For instance, jasmine cannot be distilled. The essence of this flower needs to be extracted directly from the bloom using a fatty substance. (Be aware that this is one essential oil that does contain fat and will leave an oil stain on your clothes!) Some other plants and flowers have no fragrance when they're distilled, and so extraction is the method that must be used.

When we come into contact with plant and flower essences, it is as if we are experiencing the very plants and flowers from which they were derived. As a result, these essences are very active and are capable of having profound effects on us, physically and psychologically. Essential oils are, in my mind, some of the finest substances available to us, period. Since ancient times they have been used alone, or in moisturizers, soaps, scrubs, massage oils, shampoos, conditioners, fragrances, candles, and other substances because they can boost our spirits or calm our nerves. In addition, they control impurities, are antiseptics by nature, and are great solvents. The substances that contain essential oils don't coagulate because they are solvents, which by nature dilute things. They also have a tremendous influence on our body's ability to heal. Essential oils are, of course, also a great source of fragrances, which have been added to body care products for centuries. They are natural deodorants, too. I haven't used a typical deodorant in twenty-nine years—I use essential oils on my body instead!

AROMATHERAPY: WHAT IT MEANS

As I have mentioned earlier in this book, aromatherapy is an overused, often misused term. Many companies label products with petrochemicals in them as being useful for aromatherapy and lead large numbers of people down the garden path. I can't stress enough that aromas are not truly therapeutic—to our minds or our bodies—if they are not plant-derived. When we apply the knowledge gained from studying the power of pure plant aromas over our psyches, and use it in a therapeutic way, that is what aromatherapy truly is.

Aromatherapy is actually a very ancient tradition. In my home, I have a large collection of antique incense burners from around the world that speaks to this fact. Incense was used to fight off viruses in the time of the Black Plague. People in those times also sprayed their bodies with aromatics to keep other viruses and infectious disease from invading their bodies. Ancient Egyptians used herbal oils as a skin conditioner, and employed floral aromas to calm the mind and to improve the function of various glands. The Aztecs had special vapor-bath rooms called *tmezcals*, in which a saunalike atmosphere was enhanced with the vapors of flowers and herbs. This was an accepted method of softening the skin, improving circulation, and relaxing the mind. For thousands of years, the Jews have sniffed spice boxes filled with cloves to extend into the rest of the week the happy feeling associated with the Sabbath. There is no question as to the power of aroma in affecting health and behavior. Today we are simply adding scientific corroboration to age-old practices. In studies we do at AVEDA, using machines that track brain activity and cameras which photograph a person's aura, we are able to document the effects of aromas on mood with empirical data. The more active one's brain is, the higher the vibration and the redder the aura color. The calmer one's brain is, the lower the vibration and the lighter the aura color, with a tendency toward blue and pastel shades. White is the most passive color one's aura can have. When subjects are given yin, or calming scents, to inhale, there is less tension reflected in their brain activity and their aura photographs are lighter in color. When subjects are given yang, or stimulating scents, to sniff, there is higher brain activity. When that stimulating scent is unpleasant, the aura color is closer to the highly active red.

Aromatherapy is being adopted even by practitioners of Western medicine. Today hospitals are recognizing the power of nurturing fragrances as opposed to that "hospital smell" and are diffusing essential oils on their corridors to encourage all sorts of healing. This wisdom is just beginning to

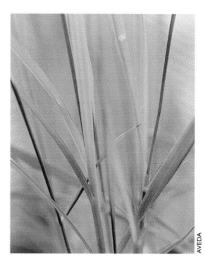

Citronella and myrtle are two of many plants that provide essential oils with wonderful effective deodorant properties.

AROMAS THAT HEAL

SPECIAL PHYSICAL CONDITIONS	ESSENTIAL OIL	
Low Vitality	basil	peppermint
	bergamot	rose
	geranium	rosemary
	lavender, spike	sandalwood
	orange	
Lower Back Pain	basil	lavender
	chamomile	peppermint
	eucalyptus	rosemary
	geranium	tea tree
	juniper	
Premenstrual Tension	bergamot	rose
	chamomile	rosemary
	clary sage	sandalwood
	geranium	ylang-ylang
	lavender	
Stress	basil	lemon
	bergamot	lemongrass
	chamomile	neroli
	clary sage	olibanum
	geranium	palmarosa
	jasmine	rosemary
	lavandin	ylang-ylang
	lavender	

SPECIAL APPLICATIONS	ESSENTIAL OIL	
Calming Effects	chamomile	neroli
	lavender	olibanum
	marjoram, sweet	rose
Energizing Effects	bergamot	pepper, black
	eucalyptus	peppermint
	lemon	rosemary
Inhalation	clove	peppermint
	eucalyptus	rosemary
	lavender	

take hold in the United States, where the Memorial Sloan-Kettering Hospital in New York started adding fragrance to reduce stress levels to rooms where MRI (magnetic resonance imaging) procedures are given. According to a 1994 report in the *Journal of Magnetic Resonance*, the group exposed to fragrance experienced 63 percent less anxiety than the control group. In Europe and Great Britain, aromatherapy is almost commonplace in hospital environments, where it is used for sedation, for pain management, for deodorization, and for general patient well-being. Perhaps this is due in part to the studies that have been conducted in that country regarding aromatherapy's effectiveness. In *Aromatherapy for Health Professionals*, by Shirley and Len Price, the authors report that in the intensive care and coronary unit of the Royal Sussex Hospital in Great Britain, aromatherapy and massage were shown to decrease blood pressure, heart rate, pain, respiratory rate, and wakefulness. Additionally, it was discovered that, although massage was beneficial, the patients who received the greatest improvements in all areas were those who were exposed to essential oils as well as massage. Similar results came from a study in London Middlesex Hospital, where massage was found to be helpful for patients in intensive care, but massage with essential oils gave enhanced and longer-lasting effects. At another British hospital, when aromas were diffused throughout the coronary care unit, there was a 71 percent reduction in anxiety levels, as compared to a 25 percent decrease in a control sample of patients who were exposed to the aromas during their stay, according to a report prepared by C. M. Harris for the Royal Shrewsbury Hospital in 1993. At a hospital in Salisbury, according to *Aromatherapy for Health Professionals*, it was found that diffused lavender relieved insomnia so well that many patients no longer needed sleeping pills. Medical schools in Germany, the United Kingdom, and the United States are beginning to teach aromatherapy to their students; and Purdue University recently added its first postgraduate course in the field. It is my hope that this will just increase the use of natural plant essences as stress relievers and sleep aids by the Western medical establishment and thereby increase every patient's comfort level.

In a related field, plant aromas are used more and more as behavior-modification tools in weight-loss programs as well. This makes a lot of sense. After all, our sense of smell is largely responsible for our sense of taste, and it has a lot to do with stimulating appetite through memory response. Just smelling a food we like can arouse a sensation of hunger within us and can even make us feel as if we are tasting that food when we're not. Therefore, aromas seem to play a big role in weight management. A psychiatrist and neurologist named Dr. Alan Hirsch did a six-month study at

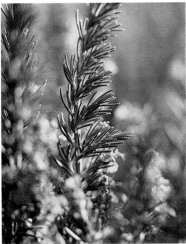

Rosemary, a powerful herb that provides relief from low vitality and lower back pain to premenstrual pain

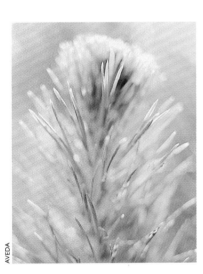

Put that coffee aside! Take a big smell of pine to get your brain moving!

the Smell and Research Foundation in Chicago on 3,190 subjects and found that by using special aroma cassettes, patients lost an average of thirty pounds each. Which fragrance worked the best in helping patients curb their cravings and overeating? Wouldn't we love to have a simple answer for that! As it turns out, the effective scents differed from case to case. The fragrances that each subject liked the best were most effective in curbing their appetite. That is why we all should explore an array of aromas to target those we like most. This involves what I call a "sensory journey." At an AVEDA store, a health food store, or an herb shop, we can sniff a wide variety of essential oils to see how we respond to various fragrances, and which ones make us feel happy. I urge you to do this and make notes of all your reactions to each essence. The scents you determine as your favorites can enhance your life by helping you accomplish your goals and savor many daily experiences more intensely.

Aromatherapy can be very personal. How we respond psychologically to different scents can be determined by our elemental makeups (or our Ayurvedic doshas), as well as by something as subjective as our memories. Even whom we choose as mates may be affected by our senses of smell. In fact, aromas have long been associated with sexual attraction in human beings, and now we know why. We're each attracted to different sorts of human body aromas based on our makeups and our personal experiences. Our sense of smell is a big component of what we call having "chemistry" with a partner. A recently discovered sex organ in the nose, called the vomeronasal organ, is a receptor for human pheromones, and the center for determining the scents in others that attract or repel us.

However, while some of our reactions to scents are quite personal, there are aromas that are known to have certain effects on emotions and behavior regardless of our experiences. Rosemary used in the workplace, for example, has been shown to aid concentration. Smart executives can diffuse certain aromas in the air in conference rooms during important meetings as a means of evoking desired responses from people. They can promote alertness in people, as well as confidence and productivity. In Japan, aromas are frequently used in offices to increase productivity and performance. They're also often used in Las Vegas casinos as a device to lure gamblers away from the quarter slot machines and toward the dollar machines. There, they tend to use sweet combinations of leafy, spicy, and fruity essences, where the top note will be pine.

How does this work? Why does simply smelling a substance change the way we act? The human brain processes fragrances on the right side, the area most concerned with emotions. Simultaneously, the olfactory receptors also transmit fragrance to the part of the brain that controls the limbic system. The limbic system triggers memory and sexual response and activates the hypothalamus, also affecting the pituitary gland, which, in turn, oversees the release of hormones from glands to organs and cells throughout the body. So the aromas we breathe in are processed by our brains and then by various other glands and organs, resulting in changes in our emotions and, ultimately, our behavior.

Using this knowledge, we can train ourselves, much like Pavlov's dog, to respond to certain aromatic stimuli, either by using the information that's already in our scent memory banks or by adding to that data. For example, if the smell of fresh lemon reminds you of the lemonade you had as a child in summer, and arouses feelings of carefree happiness that you associated with that time in your life, you can use lemon aromatics to put yourself into a relaxed, carefree state at times when you might actually have cause to be tense. Taking the process a step further, you can take any fragrance to which you are attracted and use it to teach your brain new tricks—like controlling

WAKE-UP CALL

When you're lagging at work toward the end of the morning or the end of the day, a healthy way to snap out of a lethargic daze is to diffuse some essential oils in your office. You can use a diffuser, place some oil drops in some potpourri—or even just sniff some right out of the bottle or on a handkerchief. You can use the following chart to help you decide which of the essences with stimulating and refreshing properties you'd like to use. You can also take what I call a "sensory journey," sniffing a variety of essences to identify your favorites at an AVEDA shop, health food store, or herbalist.

SPICES	CITRUS	FLOWERS	LEAVES/RESINS	ROOTS/WOODIES
clove	orange	rose	lavender	ginger
cinnamon	lemon	jasmine	peppermint	olibanum
vanilla	lime	neroli	eucalyptus	sandalwood
thyme	bergamot	ylang-ylang	sage	tea tree
rosemary	mandarin	tuberose	rosemary	bois de rose
marjoram	lemongrass	geranium	basil	cinnamon bark
coriander	citronella	lavender	neem	cinnamon leaf
				agar wood
				pine
				cedar

AROMATIC OPTIONS

Adding aroma to our lives throughout the day every day is quite a bit easier than it might seem. With a combination of the following, we can keep ourselves practically immersed in aromatic air from dawn until dusk—and even while we sleep:

- incense
- teas
- scented candles
- massage oils
- scented shampoos and cosmetics
- essential oil in the form of sprays
- diffusers
- freshly moistened potpourri
- essential oils sniffed right from the bottle, poured into the bath, or dabbed on a handkerchief

I use these things all the time, even on airplanes to pamper and protect myself against other people's germs in the recirculated air. Bear in mind, the more essential oils you combine, the greater the protection from a wide variety of bacterias, viruses, molds, and fungi.

your appetite. This works particularly well for those overeaters who often seek food to quell anxiety and bring about nurturing feelings rather than eating in response to hunger. Feeding the brain a certain nurturing smell during moments of anxiety and allowing the hungry sensation to pass is a way of training the brain to be satisfied and comforted by this bit of aromatherapy as opposed to the less healthy habit of noshing.

THE AIR THAT WE BREATHE

Knowing what we do about what a strong response our minds and bodies have to aromas, especially those derived from plants and their essences, we can enhance our lives by surrounding ourselves with the right scents at the right times, nearly all day, every day.

Optimally, aromatherapy should be a regular habit in our lives, like lifting our window shades in the morning or brushing our teeth twice a day. In addition to the wonderful psychological and emotional benefits to the use of essential oils on a daily basis, there are environmental advantages, too. Plants and their essences are great deodorizers, antiseptics, and natural air purifiers, neutralizing the noxious chemicals in our midst.

We choose the decor in our homes to please the eye, select music to invigorate or soothe the ear, prepare food to awaken our taste, and clothe our bodies in materials that are soft to the touch. In contrast, aroma seems to be a somewhat neglected aspect of our environments. But we can take a few simple steps and fill our lives with aromas to please the nose as well as the mind and spirit, and to help us nurture ourselves toward bliss.

You first must acquaint yourself with the fragrances you like, and the fragrances that have the properties to bring about the effects you desire. For starters, I recommend stopping into an AVEDA store, a health food store, or an herb shop for a sensory journey. If you buy fragrances in a health food store, beware of bottles that don't list specific oils and just say they're filled with "fragrance" or "aroma." Check for quality and authenticity, and 100-percent-pure plant essences. Today, essential oils can also be found in certain integrated medical clinics and the offices of many chiropractors, massage therapists, and dermatologists. You'll want to find both energizing and calming fragrances of which you are fond. If you don't particularly like the oils I recommend, simply choose another stimulating or calming essence you do enjoy for my recommendations below.

The next step is to get the equipment necessary to fill the air around you with aroma. You can employ everything from the simplest handkerchief to the most complex timed diffuser to help you scent your world. Here are some methods to choose from:

▶ Use a diffuser with a timer to help you wake up in the morning. Instead of the sound of an alarm, you can be gently aroused by a whiff of citrus oils.

▶ Place simple ceramic ring diffusers above the lightbulbs in the lamps in your home and office. The heat from the bulb sparks the diffusion of the fragrance.

▶ Get special, small diffusers designed for use in cars and offices so that you can be surrounded by the aromas you love wherever you go—and be calm even in a traffic jam.

▶ Keep spray bottles filled with delicious combinations of essential oils that you love nearby you at home and at work.

▶ Spray your favorite oil or combination of oils onto your linen or onto your pillow; surround yourself and sleep with the calming scents you love.

▶ Carry little bottles of your favorite combinations with you to sniff as you need to—perhaps in the middle of the workday when your energy lags—or to pour onto tissues or handkerchiefs for sniffing.

▶ Place a few drops of essential oil in a bath, or even under a running shower—a great way to enhance the ritual of bathing with aroma.

▶ Burn candles to add the aromas you love to your environment, during meditation or mirroring, or when just relaxing. Be sure to use candles made with a high percentage of natural beeswax as opposed to petrochemical wax. Synthetic candles pollute when they're manufactured and when they're burned. Beeswax candles actually help to purify the air when burned. And, of course, never leave burning candles unattended, or you might not have a place to perform any of your new habits!

AROMATIC HEAVEN, 24/7

Here's a little schedule suggesting the ways in which we can keep our aromatherapy going all day long:

▶ Use a timed diffuser to give off energizing fragrances to wake you up and keep it going until you leave the house. Or, spray a mist of energizing oils to wake your mind up after your alarm goes off.

▶ Perform self-massage with a composition containing energizing essential oils. You leave this on through your morning exercise regimen.

» Shower with cleansers, shampoo, conditioner, and other products made with essential oils, and drop some potent oils into the shower basin.

» Splash your body with fragrances you love, as perfume and as deodorant.

» Burn incense or a fragrant beeswax candle as you do your meditation and mirroring.

» Drink an aromatic tea with breakfast.

» Clean your home with cleansers that contain essential oils.

» Diffuse stimulating or calming fragrances in the car. Or, if you take mass transit, sniff a bottle of oils or a tissue with a few drops of oil on it.

» Diffuse oils in the office, or add them to potpourri.

» Take a walk among trees and flowers during lunch, and benefit from aromatherapy for free!

» Sniff a tissue dipped in essential oils to restore energy or to stave off the 4 P.M. blood-sugar-drop junk-food cravings.

» Diffuse calming fragrances in the car on your way home.

» Diffuse some calming fragrances at home, and keep them going through the night.

» Drink an aromatic tea after dinner.

» Take a bicycle ride and enjoy the smell of the grass and foliage along whatever path you take.

» Take a relaxing bath with fragrant, calming essential oils.

» Exchange massages with your partner, or do another self-massage, using calming oils that you love.

» Spray your sheets with your favorite bedtime scents.

» Sleep the night away with a diffuser timed to burn calming fragrances until it's time for the energizing scents of morning.

A ROAD MAP OF THE SENSORY JOURNEY

The fragrances that will have the most profound positive effects on each person are the fragrances that person likes. But, as I explained earlier, some fragrances have certain properties that affect us independently of our sense memories and our feelings.

In choosing the aromas we prefer for each purpose—invigorating, calming, etc.—it helps to know the characteristics of some of the plants and their essences. You can use the following as a guide when you visit a shop where you can test several scents.

Sunrise

Among the refreshing and balancing fragrances that are recommended for waking up the morning are these: tangerine, orange, bergamot, rosemary, eucalyptus, lemon, lime, jasmine, rose, pine, and lavender. Lavender is actually a good weekend waker-upper, because it doesn't make you too "zingy."

Avoiding Road Rage

In the car, lavender is an excellent balancing oil, it can energize without being too stimulating. Rosemary is a good concentrating oil; it can help you find your car in a crowded lot at the end of the day.

Getting Going

For those of us who experience some anxiety at the beginning of the workday, geranium is a fragrance that promotes peacefulness. It's like Prozac for the nose. Peppermint is a good way to refresh and energize when lunch is still another hour or so away. A combination of lavender and rosemary will help us to concentrate in a relaxed way. A combination of olibanum and frankincense will enhance your creativity.

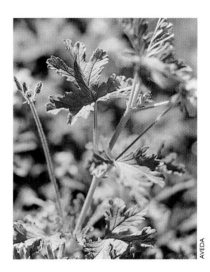

A bit of geranium's soothing smell can help you ease into the day.

The 4 P.M. Blahs

When the blood sugar crashes, it's a good idea to breathe in lavender, rosemary, or a combination of both, depending on your personal taste.

Homeward Bound

Cinnamon is a nice fragrance for the ride home. It will hold us over until dinner, relax us, and refresh us.

Back at the Ranch

Instead of a glass of wine, why not unwind with the fragrance of a vanilla-scented candle or incense? This is a favorite fragrance among children. Tangerine and rose are lovely for this rewelcoming-to-the-home time. After dinner, some jasmine will help everyone relax and get ready for sleep.

Adults Only

Ylang-ylang and sandalwood are known to have aphrodisiac effects . . . in case anyone is interested.

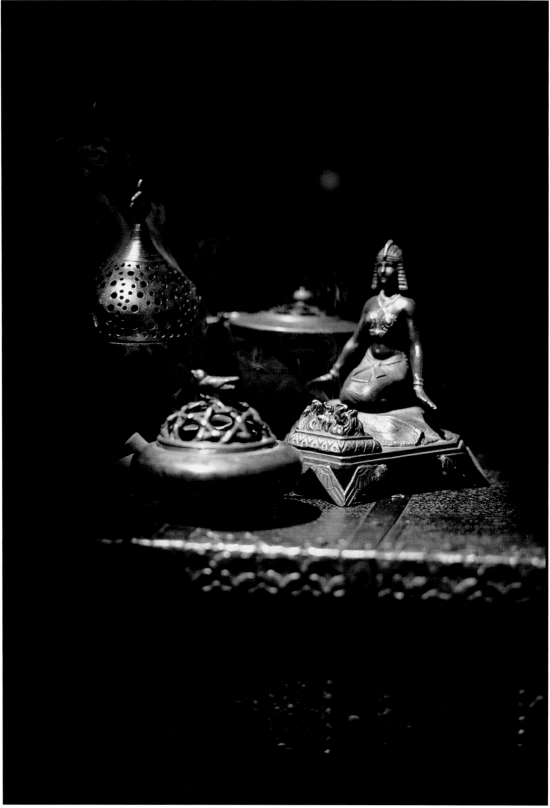

Day Is Done

Evening Relaxation

*In her starry shade of dim and solitary loveliness, I learn
the language of another world.*

—LORD BYRON

T HE SUN SETS, THE DAY FADES, AND IT'S TIME TO RELAX.
Our work is behind us—or it should be.

Winding down is not a matter of laziness, it is an essential
part of a balanced day and life. Most of us have established
ways of relaxing. They come naturally to us at this point. There
are many people, though, who really don't know how to taper off their
activity as the day comes to a close. They need constantly to be doing
things and are seemingly unable to be still, even at the end of a long workday. They don't realize that it's important to make time in our schedules for
leisure and repose so that we can prepare ourselves for quality sleep and
reserve energy for the next day. It's also key for our minds to get a break after
several hours of working, commuting, and coping with stresses that are out
of our control.

Shifting into a lower gear as the evening appears is both natural and necessary. But it is important to note that there are some ways of approaching it
that are nurturing to us, and some that are not. For example, no one needs
to tell you that being a couch potato—spending evening after evening just

flipping the channels on your television set, snacking, and doing hardly anything else—has little benefit for mind, body, and spirit. It may feel relaxing at the moment, but in the long run, you'll become more stressed out from the lack of motion and lack of attention to your greater intentions. That's not to say you should never watch television or go to the movies. But on a regular basis, eating a quiet dinner, meditating and reflecting on the day that has just passed, taking an evening walk or bike ride, and participating in partner massage are components of a sort of very relaxing routine, which can help you stay in touch with and move further toward your goals over time.

DINING ROOM

Do you eat your dinner on the run, standing at the counter and reading the paper? There are people who actually eat "dinner" standing in front of an open refrigerator, grabbing what they can before they move on to whatever activity they've planned next. Lots of people eat in front of the television, or save their important family discussions and arguments for this time of night.

As I've said in previous chapters, eating time is for eating, and eating only. Some pleasant conversation is a nice complement to a good meal, as is some nice music along with an aromatic candle. But activities that do not please or awaken the senses can only detract from our eating experiences.

Being mindful of our food, how it feels and tastes and smells, is an important part of our self-nurturing experience. In addition, digestion can be disrupted by stress. You can discuss the bills or your in-laws either before or after dinner if they're on your mind. But when you sit down to eat, the meal should be a pleasant, comforting experience that is part of a positive routine.

Eating dinner in a calm, mindful manner can arouse feelings of gratitude for all that is good in your life. It's a great time and place to give thanks to your partner, your family, your friends, and whatever divine spirit with which you identify. At the end of the day, it's nice to give a prayer of thanks, silently or out loud, in whatever language you know.

KICKING BACK

When the evening rolls around, I enter what I call a letting-go mode. I simply don't want to do much. Rather than being highly active at this point in the day, I switch gears and become an observer, of myself and the people and things in my life. This is the beginning of the inventory process.

I try to apply mindfulness to all that I do—and don't do—when I return home from a day at the office. It begins as soon as I get home. There's actually a *plan* to my relaxation. After I've unwound a bit and done some meditation and mirroring, I try to organize an evening schedule for myself and my partner when she gets home. I try to plot some bliss for the evening. I think it can be very romantic, and very nurturing to both partners, if you plan evenings out once in a while.

Of course, if I am planning events that include my partner, I must listen to her desires, too. If I have planned an evening of dancing but she is too exhausted from a long day and a long ride home, I need to adjust my formula for the evening. But first I need to listen to my own heart to discover my threshold for late-day activity.

It's a good idea to do your evening meditation and mirroring in the earlier part of the night. You can learn from your silence and stillness just what you're game for, in terms of your energy and your mood that night. There might be nights when a quiet dinner and massage are all you can handle, and others when you'd like to dance and rejoice before you turn in. I also just find that twilight provides good lighting and quiet for meditation and mirroring. I do my best meditation then, and also just before dawn. Once you've meditated and reflected on the day behind you, you can create a scheme for the rest of your evening.

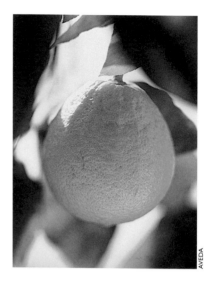

NIGHT MOVES

Although it might seem like an oxymoron, there is such a thing as purposeful relaxation. That would include anything that you find both calming and consciousness-raising. We can be placid while also being aware through all our senses. It is this awareness that keeps us in touch with our true emotions and intentions and helps us to stay on track with our positive, nurturing routines. Among the practices that might fit the bill are these:

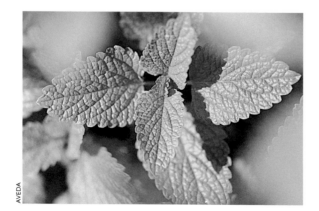

*B*ergamot *(above) and melissa (left) are two calming oils that are perfect for an evening massage.*

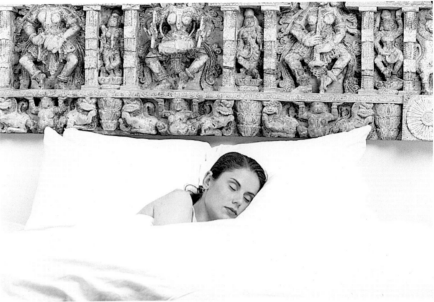

A bit of lavender in the bedroom will provide a scent that can help ease you into a deep, peaceful sleep.

HORST RECHELBACHER

- breathing exercises to lower the heart rate, such as exhaling twice as long as you inhale, and being aware of the slower pace
- listening to some music that you love, but that isn't too stimulating
- dimming the lights
- reading
- performing yoga or tai chi, but not vigorously
- doing gentle aerobic exercise, such as walking, biking, swimming, or slow dancing
- enjoying aromatherapy, in the form of a candle at dinner; an warm, aromatic bath; or some massage oils such as soothing and calming bergamot or melissa
- meditating and mirroring, reviewing what happened all day, and making a plan for tomorrow from what you've assessed
- trading massages with your partner

All of these practices will allow you to be calm and mellow, while also arousing your senses and encouraging mental and spiritual consciousness. This is the kind of consciousness that leads over time to genuine peace of mind. You can engage in all or just some of these practices each evening. There will be times when you want a night full of adventures, and others when you just need to be still. Listen to your heart in your meditation and mirroring, and it will tell you what kind of evening to plan.

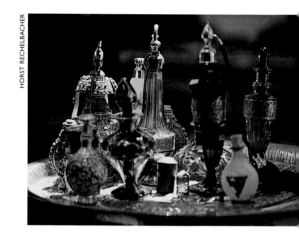

Clean and Simple

Cleansing Body and Mind

God can never be realized by one who is not pure of heart. Self-purification therefore must mean purification in all walks of life. And purification being highly infectious, purification of oneself usually leads to the purification of one's surroundings.

—MAHATMA GANDHI

THE SAYING THAT CLEANLINESS IS NEXT TO GODLINESS could have its roots in any number of the world's cultures. Through the ages, outer cleanliness has been associated with inner purification by many. Bathing and dousing with water have been parts of ceremonial rituals including baptisms and the monthly purification of Jewish women in a *mikvah* pool. Because we now recognize how strongly mind, body, and spirit are bound, we realize how true it is that when we feel clean on the outside, we are more likely to feel clean on the inside, and vice versa.

Ritual baths have also been associated with beauty throughout history. Royalty in Indonesia used to beautify themselves for ceremonious occasions with a series of cleansing treatments called a *lulur* bath. They'd soak in tubs filled with fragrant water and frangipani flowers, then have exfoliating treatments with sea salt, and finish with a soothing bath of yogurt to soften the skin. One of Cleopatra's beauty secrets is said to have been bathing in cow's milk and mountain waters containing the essences of herbs and flowers.

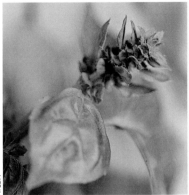

Basil's not just for pasta! Its essential oil added to your bath or shower will warm you up on a cold winter night.

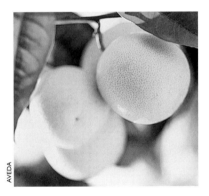

To cool down after a summer day or workout, add petitgrain to your soak.

Whether or not an hour in a hot tub can transform us into perfectly pure and stunning creatures, our cleansing rituals can have a profound effect on how we feel, inside and out. We all know the restorative magic of a soak in a fragrant bubble bath if the aroma is one we deeply love, or a soothing, warm shower. Clearly, the effects of bathing are not limited to the physical; we are affected mentally and spiritually as well, especially if we take steps to make our cleansing rituals very personal. We can enhance our daily washing routine by choosing favorite scents, lighting, and sounds, or just by bringing a new frame of mind to it.

Of course, outer cleansing is already part of everyone's daily routine. It's not a new ritual. But perhaps not all of us have looked at bathing and cleansing as a therapeutic ritual or nurturing habit. We can adjust our perspective on this, simply by adding a second one. This simple change of mind can provide aromatherapeutic body cleansing, with calming cleansers and oils, to the end of the day.

STEEPED IN SCENT-IMENT

Bathing can be so much more than just a skin-washing, deodorizing endeavor. It is an opportunity for you to incorporate aromatherapy in a very relaxing, comforting, womblike environment.

You can practice aromatherapy as you wash, whether you take a bath or a shower. There are several categories of products that you can include in your body-cleansing practice to add beneficial fragrances. Soap, body wash, shampoo, conditioner, invigorating scrubs, bath salts, and bath oils are all available with essential oils in them. AVEDA makes a whole array of these products in both calming and energizing formulas.

You can also make your own. Herbal essences and distilled oils from flowers can easily be combined with natural detergents like castille soap to make excellent foaming bath formulas. Most of the ingredients necessary for homemade versions can be found in health food stores. Just make sure you choose a reputable store, and ask whether the preparations you're receiving have maximum purity and potency. It's just as important that you find the essential oil or combination of oils that raises your spirit. The last chapter of this book includes some recipes for all sorts of products with essential oils that you might want to try.

As far as bath oils are concerned, they can be as simple as pure essential oils. You can add them—just a few drops—to a hot bath, or place them in the basin of the shower stall or tub during a shower. As the water hits the oil or oils on the floor during a shower, it disperses and diffuses them into your shower steam.

Essential oils can have yin, relaxing and cooling properties, or yang, stimulating and warming properties. Essences with yin properties help us to unwind and are especially useful for the end of the day when we want to prepare for restful sleep. Essences with yang properties help to invigorate and stimulate us, making these oils perfect for the morning when we need to get energized to meet the day ahead.

Essential oils can also help us control our reactions to our climate. By using yin essences in summer, we can help our bodies stay cool; by using yang essences in winter, we can help our bodies stay warm.

Here's a list of some essential oils and their properties. You can use them alone, but for bathing purposes, it's often beneficial to use them in combination because then we reap more antibacterial, antifungal, antiviral, and antiyeast benefits. The key is figuring out just how much of each to use. Just a few tiny drops are usually quite potent. In fact, it can be dangerous to use too much of some essential oils, as they can be very active on our skin, causing sensitivity, irritation, or burning. Proper dilution is very important. Make sure you learn the proper base-to-oil ratio from whoever sells essential oils to you. AVEDA has several ready-made dilutions, in the form of perfumes, or what we call "Pure-fumes."

In addition to these essences' wonderful aromas and mood-changing benefits through olfactory memory response—which activates an internal chemistry that turns the body into its own pharmacist—they can also have wonderful direct influences on the skin and muscles. The combination of warm water and active, energizing essential oils can soothe sore muscles after a long day or a hard workout, and reduce swelling of minor sprains. If you have a specific area you want to soothe, you can rub some oils into them before stepping into the bath or shower. This ensures the oil's deep penetration. With the heat of the bath, they are sure to soak to the core of your aching muscles and work their rejuvenation magic there. These oils you rub directly on your skin should be mixed with a base oil, like jojoba, coconut, sesame, avocado, hazelnut, walnut, grape seed, or even olive. Undiluted, the essential oils are too strong for direct application on your body.

YIN
(relaxing and cooling)

eucalyptus

Siberian fir

cypress

camphor

rose

chamomile

ylang-ylang (geranium)

lemon

petitgrain (leaf/root of
   orange)

mandarin

citronella

lime

YANG
(stimulating and warming)

cedarwood

frankincense

myrrh

sandalwood

lavender

jasmine

neroli (orange blossom)

bergamot

peppermint

marjoram

fennel

basil

wintergreen

olibanum (frankincense)

BRAIN WASHING

While you're in the tub or the shower, if you have the time, you can use these precious moments of comfort to further reinforce your mind-body-

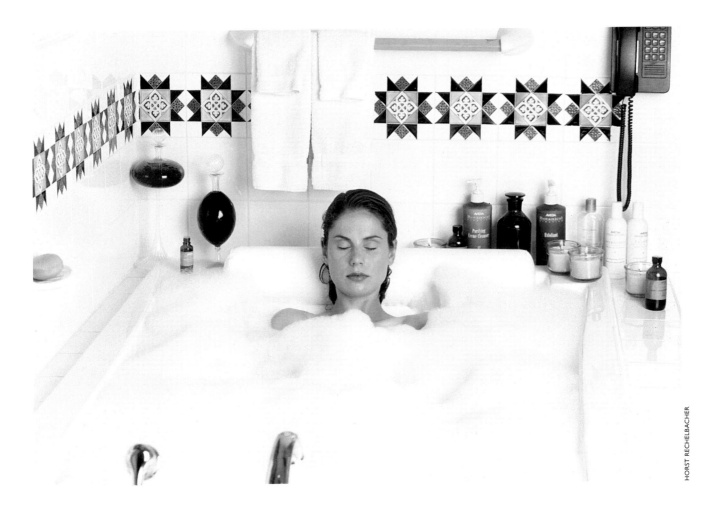

HORST RECHELBACHER

An aromatherapy bath does more than clean; it rejuvenates the mind and spirit as well.

spirit connection. While you wash on the outside, also cleanse your mind of negative thoughts. Refill your mind with positive thoughts. If you are so inclined, you'll find the bathtub is a nice place to do your mirroring, affirmations, and even meditation. The combination of the water's soothing warmth and the effects of the essential oils will put you in a receptive state for inner reflection and contemplation.

Of course, this is just one of many places you can practice your inner work. In the subchapter "Reflections," I discuss mirroring and meditation and how to create places of sanctuary for them. I just suggest this here to help alert you to the many possible ways you can enhance your daily cleansing routine. Remember the holistic nature of our existence and the many layers and aspects of our lives we can enhance and address quite simply. A subtle shift in our mind-set, an awareness of our complex natures, and a focus on self-nurturing are all ways in which we can create a life of meaning and depth that brings us closer to the fulfillment we are seeking. Every small move we make toward recognizing the world and all the life it supports as important elements in our own lives gives our existence the meaning that energizes and excites us.

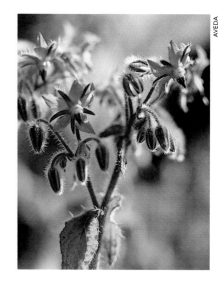

To Love, Honor, Cherish, and Massage

I will reveal to you a love potion without medicine, without herbs, without any witch's magic; if you want to be loved, then love.

—HECATON OF RHODES

HOSE OF US WHO HAVE PARTNERS—HUSBANDS, WIVES, girlfriends, boyfriends, or significant others, if you prefer—are very lucky. We have live-in masseurs!

Forget about the notion of massage as a frivolous indulgence or a treat for rare occasions. We all need to get massaged every day to maintain optimal health and happiness. Those of us who don't have partners can practice self-massage more than once a day. But those with a partner are doubly blessed. With that other person comes the opportunity to both give and receive regular loving, healing touch.

There is evidence that massaging promotes healing in many ways. It helps our bodies' many systems to release toxins, increase blood flow, and deliver nutrients to all parts of the body. The soothing touch it involves helps us to feel connected and loved. Daily partner massage helps us to keep the flow of life energy and healing energy stronger and more consistent within ourselves. As I will discuss in the chapter on healing, we all have the

IN THE MOOD

Before you and your partner exchange massages, you should each get into the right frame of mind for nurturing and being nurtured. Following are some of the steps you can take:

▸ Create a boundary between yourselves and the rest of your lives. Turn off the television, the ringer on your phone, the computer, and any other potential sources of distraction or disturbance.

▸ Maybe take a warm, aromatic bath or shower beforehand, to begin the relaxation process.

▸ Do some diaphragmatic breathing exercises to relax your breath, whether you are about to give or receive a massage. Both partners must be in a peaceful state for the massages to be mutually satisfying.

▸ Light beeswax candles scented with plant-based aromas.

▸ Diffuse throughout the room essential oils that you both love.

▸ Play soothing music or tapes of nature sounds such as the crashing of ocean waves.

▸ Set your lighting so that it is gentle on the eyes.

ability to transfer healing energy from ourselves to others, and to direct that energy to the places where it is most needed. There are also aromatherapeutic and physiological benefits to be gained by both the masseur and "maseuee" when you mix a massage base with a few drops of active plant essences that you both feel totally nurtured by.

When we massage each other, we bring about a vibrational exchange that promotes oneness between two people, strengthening our relationships and helping us to improve communication. Massage is just another way of experiencing and amplifying our connection to another. If our relationships with our partners are to be successful, we need to maintain a constant exchange of energy, love, touch, and nurturance. This is a symbiotic relationship; we are interdependent. As with any of the relationships in our lives, we need to sustain our partners as they need to sustain us. If our intentions are just to do for ourselves and not to consider our partners, then we will never achieve oneness. But we should also not forget that it takes more than touch communication to repair a relationship. As with everything in life, it requires a holistic approach, involving with both partners' minds, bodies, and spirits.

We also need to practice self-love in order to be truly available for our partners. Oneness starts with the self. The biggest disease in the world really is loneliness. When we are one with ourselves, we are not lonely and we are more likely to choose partners with whom we can have nurturing relationships.

This process of two becoming one works only when there is no expectation, just giving to each other unconditionally. That includes giving loving touch. Each partner should give the other a massage each day. (George Burns had a massage a day for most of his adult life, and he lived to be one hundred! He had his cigars and his whiskey, but he counteracted that with daily exercise, massage, and plenty of laughter.) That massage can last for as little as ten minutes or as long as an hour, varying each day, and depending upon the availability of time. If you don't have a lot of time one night, don't be discouraged and throw in the towel—use what little time you do have to exchange mini-massages.

Bear in mind that when we give a massage we also get a massage— and not just because we're taking turns. The masseur benefits from a massage, too. That is in keeping with a basic law of the universe: Giving is receiving. You cannot give without receiving some benefit. And you can't receive without giving, either—even if you're just providing the other person with the satisfaction of having freely and openly given something to you.

PERSONALIZED TOUCH

We each prefer different degrees of pressure in massage. Some of us like to have every inch of our muscles intensely kneaded, and others prefer just a light sweeping of the hands over the skin. What's the *right* way to give a massage? The way the person wants to receive it. Here are some guidelines to keep in mind regarding partner massage:

▸ Everyone has his or her own threshold for massage pressure. Each partner should respect the other's preferences and indulge them.

▸ Speak up about your massage preferences. Partner massage is meant to facilitate communication.

▸ Before giving a massage, connect with the life force within you through introspection and breathing exercises. This will help you to project this energy and direct it toward the regions where your partner needs healing. This is the basis of the Japanese tradition of healing touch called Reiki.

▸ Always give a massage with love. The intent is an important factor in getting positive results. Massaging with anger can lead to physical and/or emotional injury.

▸ Always massage toward the heart.

PROFESSIONAL SECRETS REVEALED!

Following are diagrams and instructions for massaging your partner's body. In addition to the techniques here, you'll find instruction for healing reflexology massage—performed on the soles of the feet—in Chapter 9. That's a massage that should be given about once a month, or as needed, for healing.

Make sure you choose essential oils to which each partner responds well, both to the touch and through the sense of smell. Go on a sensory journey together sometime to figure out which ones those are.

TERMS OF ENDEARMENT

Here are some terms you'll need to learn if you're going to engage in partner massage.

▸ Effleurage—a gentle, stroking motion

▸ Petrissage—a pulsating motion using intermittent pressure

▸ Kneading—an intense, circular motion that burrows into the muscles

Apply a generous amount of your partner's warm, customized massage blend using a press, release, and slide movement; beginning at the décolleté, work up to the forehead following the lymphatic flow.

Position hands on the décolleté, forming a triangle with thumbs resting on clavicle. Ask your partner to take three diaphragmatic breaths. Lean forward and apply pressure as he or she exhales.

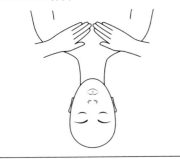

Perform three upper body hugs. Effleurage across décolleté, down the inside of the arm, around the elbow, and up the back of the arms to occipital, and massage in circular movements.

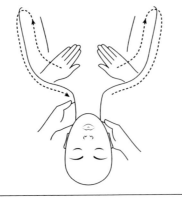

Turn the head to the left. Using the right hand with an effleurage movement, slide over the side of neck, over front of deltoid to elbow, up the back of the arm and trapezius, ending at occipital with circular movement. Return to beginning position.

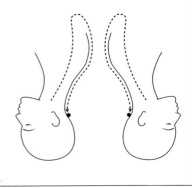

Transition to trapezius and massage with thumbs.

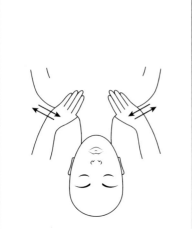

Slide hands around shoulders and massage trapezius with flat fingers and/or knuckling. Transition to center of the décolleté.

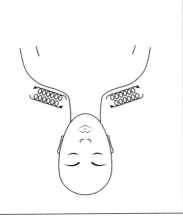

Stimulate the point found between the breasts. With four flat fingers, slowly pump out to axilla and continue to pump at axilla.

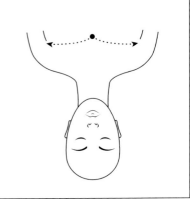

Stimulate next pressure point one inch above the previous point along midline and continue to pump with flat finger out to axilla. Continue to pump at axilla.

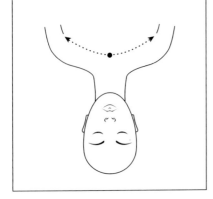

Stimulate the two points found between the first and second rib (these points are separated by a distance about the width of the neck). Pump out to the axilla.

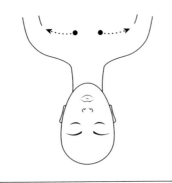

Stimulate the two lung points found one inch below the clavicle and six inches exterior to midline; pump down to axilla.

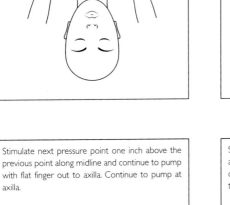

Return to center of décolleté and pump out to axilla. Continue in this fashion until you have covered the décolleté thoroughly. Spend extra concentrated time pumping at the axilla area.

With thumb and middle finger, pinch the clavicle. Starting from the midline, pinch and slide along clavicle to shoulders. Pump to axilla.

Transition around shoulders to either side of the spine. Slide down either side of the spine to the two points on the back, opposite the breast points. Using a pumping and lifting movement, move up either side of the spine to occipital ridge. Locate the point in the hollow at center of occipital ridge and stimulate the pressure point.

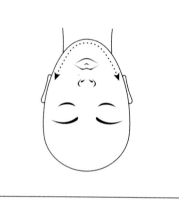

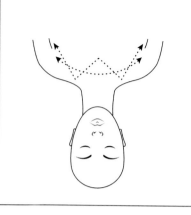

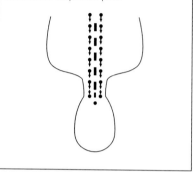

Turn head to the left. Stimulate the point to the right of center point. Using the back of fingers, pump down the back of the neck. Pump several times in the hollow of clavicle. Stimulate next pressure point along the occipital ridge, and pump down to clavicle. Continue to pump down the neck, clearing that side completely. Repeat on the left side, starting at the pressure point just left of center.

Return the head to center. Place flat fingers along the chin; continue to pump laterally along the jaw and out to the ears.

Pump the earlobes; pinch up and down the outer ridge, then the middle ridge. Ask your partner for permission to stimulate the inner part of the ear.

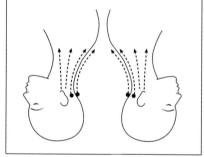

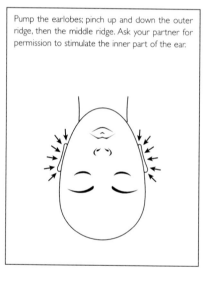

Scissors the ears between the index and ring fingers. Slide back and forth with firm pressure.

Stimulate pressure points found at the notch located about one finger's width anterior to the earlobe. Pump to behind the ears and down the neck, pumping several times at the clavicle. Continue to pump down to axilla.

Stimulate the pressure point below the lower lip. Pump to earlobes. Continue pumping down the neck using the back of fingers. Pump at hollow of clavicle.

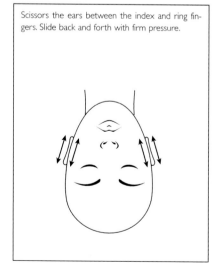

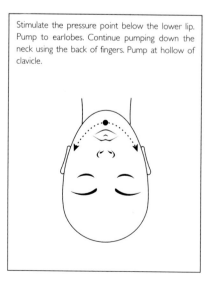

Stimulate the pressure point between nose and upper lip. Pump out to middle of ear.

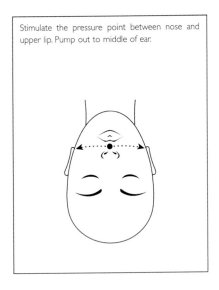

Stimulate the points located on either side of the flair of the nostrils. Pump out to the pressure point at the zygomatic arch.

Stimulate the points, then continue to pump along the zygomatic ridge to earlobes.

Place fingers at either side of the bridge of the nose. Pump the sides of the nose to the next points found at the end of the cartilage. You will feel a small indentation. Stimulate those points and pump out to midear.

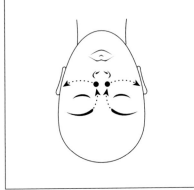

Reposition fingers at the bridge of the nose. Pump down to the points below the orbital bone. Slowly perform small, gentle pumps laterally along the orbital bone draining under the eye to the hairline. Using flat fingers, pump down to the mandible. Using the backs of fingers, slowly pump down the neck to clavicle. Pump several times.

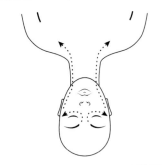

Stimulate the points at the beginning of the eyebrows. Pinch laterally along eyebrows to the temples. Reposition fingers at the center of forehead above eyebrows and pump out toward temple area to hairline. Continue to return to midline and pump out until entire forehead is covered.

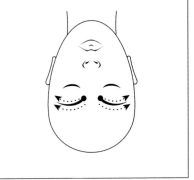

On the final forehead movement, pump all the way down the perimeter to clavicle. Pump at clavicle and continue to pump down to axilla.

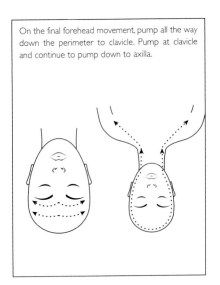

Return to forehead and pump back to crown along the midline.

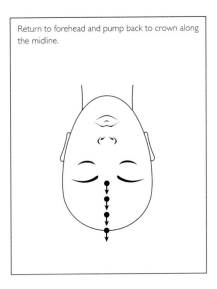

Apply a composition to the entire scalp. Using all fingers, vigorously massage the entire scalp with a rapid back and forth "shampooing" method. Continue for about one minute.

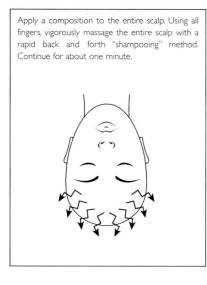

Perform therapeutic brushing—working in all directions to stimulate scalp and distribute composition.

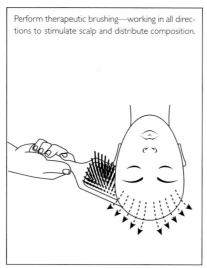

Perform pressure-point massage—working from the hairline to the crown in pie-shaped sections; press the scalp between your thumbs to increase blood flow to the scalp.

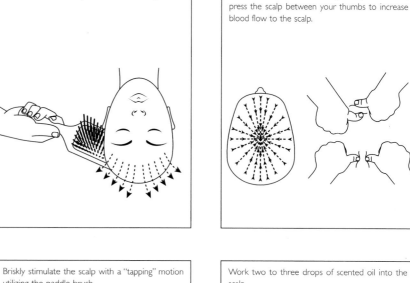

Gently pull the hair at the roots. Brush hair thoroughly.

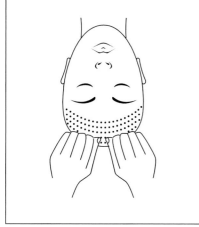

Briskly stimulate the scalp with a "tapping" motion utilizing the paddle brush.

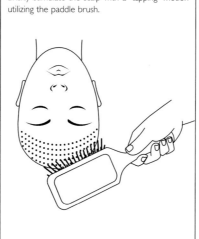

Work two to three drops of scented oil into the scalp.

Wash hands thoroughly before continuing the massage.

THE ARM AND HAND MASSAGE

Apply massage product to hand and arm with alternating movements from wrist to shoulder, covering the entire arm.

Work from wrist to elbow using circular movements to begin releasing tense areas.

Rotate the wrist several times in one direction, then the other. Work the palm using the thumb between the first and second metacarpals (thumb and index fingers) using a slow effleurage motion starting at the base of the hand moving toward the base of the fingers. Repeat this motion between the second and third, third and fourth, and fourth and fifth metacarpals starting at the base of the hand moving toward the base of the fingers.

Massage the palm using circular friction motions with your thumb. Begin at the base of the thumb and work up toward the base of the index finger. Continue to work across toward the fourth finger and down the side to the heel completing at the center of the palm.

Turn hand over starting at the wrist, using an effleurage movement. Work toward the fingers in between the digits.

Starting with the thumb, use a pinch, release, and slide motion from the base to the tip, covering the sides, top, and bottom of the digit. Complete each digit by stimulating the four pressure points located at the tip, and finish with a gentle pull.

Stimulate the pressure point located between the thumb and index finger.

Massage from the wrist to elbow and elevate the arm over your partner's head. Continue using circular movements over the triceps to release tension from the back of the arm.

Gently stretch the arm above your partner, straight out, and down along your partner's side. Place the arm back in its normal relaxed position, and finish with several sweeping movements.

Repeat sequence on the other hand and arm.

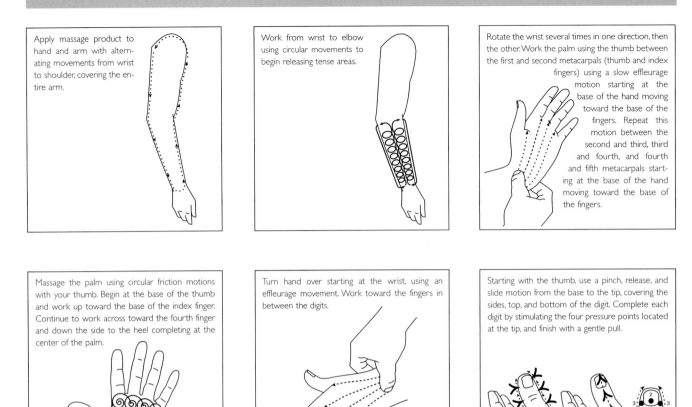
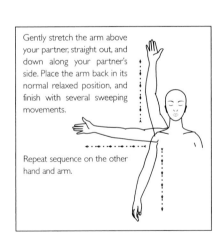

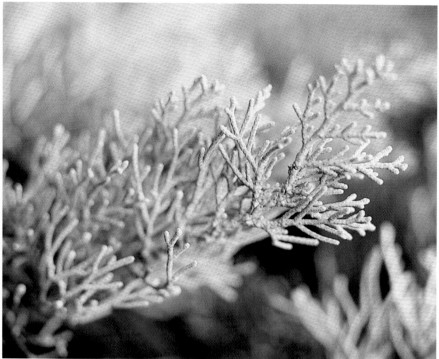

For a stimulating massage, try adding cypress oil to your massage oil base.

EQUAL TIME

I've talked a lot in this book about the importance of planning. That applies to partner massage as well. Figure it into the scheme of your evening so that this very valuable practice doesn't fall by the wayside. No matter how busy your life gets, create some amount of time for this regularly. Also make sure you leave time for switching turns with your partner, and for a gentle transition as you exchange roles, going from masseur to masseuee, or vice versa.

You also need to allow time for each of you to hone your massage techniques. Keep the instructions I've provided handy in the beginning. The more you practice, the better you will get at nurturing each other through touch. Make sure that you listen to each other as you speak up about which motions feel good and which cause discomfort.

Once you've begun trading massages with your partner, you're likely to look forward to this practice each day. You will both look and feel healthier. And your relationship will benefit, too. Once you've begun to enjoy the pleasures of regular massage with a partner, you'll want to share its benefits with all those who are special in your life. Be generous!

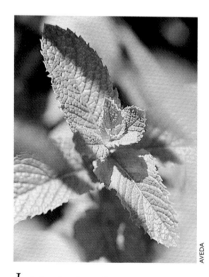

Indulge in the calming essence of a spearmint rubdown.

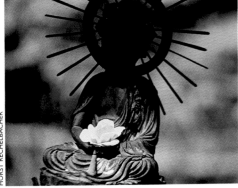

Reflections

Mirroring and Meditation

Close your eyes and you will see clearly.
Cease to listen and you will hear truth.
Be silent and your heart will sing.
Seek no contact and you will find union.
Be still and you will move on the tide of the spirit.
Be gentle and you will need no strength.
Be patient and you will achieve all things.
Be humble and you will remain entire.

—ANONYMOUS TAOIST POEM

WHEN YOU LOOK AT YOURSELF IN THE MIRROR, WHAT do you see? When you look at yourself through your own internal vision mirror, what do you see?

Maybe you haven't taken a good look at yourself in the mirror—the external mirror or the internal mirror—in some time. When you're in a mode of acting out of rote, without mindfulness or consciousness, you tend to avoid the mirrors on the wall and in the mind. But taking inventory of ourselves—of all the sectors of our beings—is a very important tool in creating and maintaining a set of nurturing daily practices. This self-analysis is the place where we begin to heal from all the stresses in our lives. It is where we learn to forgive ourselves, let go of our anger at ourselves and others, and allow our souls to mend. It is the place where we choose how to mend. Mirroring is a key to improving our lives and attaining our goals. It is a direct way to consciousness, which is a clear path to the zone of bliss. It is a process we need to confront daily, fearlessly and lovingly. Mirroring is also a good precursor to meditation. In this chapter, I will discuss both mirroring and meditation—what they are, why we do them, and ways to go about them.

MIRROR, MIRROR . . .

Mirroring should be a daily practice, and under the best of circumstances, it is advisable to do it three times a day—in the morning before or after meditation, in the afternoon at work, and at the end of the day, before bedtime. It also can be done on a grander scale, on a weekly, monthly, and/or annual basis, and can be combined with fasting and silence as part of an inner-cleansing ritual. In Chapter 9, I'll discuss these special, occasional practices.

What exactly is mirroring? It is several things. It is a one-on-one interview with the self, a question-and-answer session in which we take mindful note of all the things we have been doing and all the things we want to achieve. It is an evaluation session in which we consider those habits of ours that are causing us pain, and those that are helping us grow and get closer to bliss. It is what is known in televised sports as instant replay, a chance to review the past so that we can learn and make better plans for the future.

Mirroring can take many forms. It can be a simple matter of making time to be alone to reflect on what has taken place so far in the day, and to adjust our game plan for the rest of the day. It can come in the form of journal writing, or list making. Diaries are very useful for keeping us conscious and focused. We can make lists of positives and negatives in our lives, or sources of pain and bliss, and apply the law of cause and effect to figure out which things we need to change or adjust. Writing down the things we don't like about our choices thus far is just as important as writing down the things we do like. Making lists of goals is another way to approach mirroring.

I like the idea of keeping in touch with our goals or our intentions. We need to have goals in our lives, for both the near and far future. We need to plan our lives. Of course, we also need to remain flexible and adjust our goals as our lives change. When we are too rigid about our goals, we can lose out on opportunities that might be even better for us than what we had planned for ourselves. So have goals, and then release them in meditation.

Just because we are not too attached to our goals doesn't mean we can't remind ourselves of them, though. We can keep a frame on our nightstand filled with our goals, which we can change as we see fit. We can write our goals on the cover of our diary or journal. Staying conscious of our

THE MAN IN THE MIRROR

I started mirroring in 1968, the year I learned to meditate, and it changed my life in ways I could never have imagined. In fact, I attribute the success and growth of my business to this practice of reflecting on my life and my rituals and continuously adjusting them based on what I've discovered in daily, weekly, seasonal, and annual mirroring. Prior to my first mirroring sessions, I didn't even realize that I was living my life without any vision. Without vision, there is no growth; and without mirroring and goal setting, there is no vision.

It was so simple. I just began writing down observations about my days and how I lived them, noticing, in every aspect of my life, which of my habits were working for me and which weren't. Then I began writing down goals. Writing them down made them somehow real and helped to keep them in my consciousness at all times. As a result, I have made all of my goals manifest. That's not to say that I am done with all I ever wished to do. The achievement of every one of my goals spawned new ones, which required new reflection on how to achieve them.

GOING BACK TO
THE MIRROR

None of us is perfect. Often when we embark on a new regimen—whether it be a new diet, an exercise regimen, or a holistic set of rituals—we begin with lots of enthusiasm and energy, which we later find difficult to sustain. It is so easy to get discouraged as soon as we fall off course, and then to give up our new habits altogether. But just because we lost our way for a while doesn't mean we can't find our way back once again to a healthy, nurturing path.

I have gone back and forth many times with my own practice of healthy daily rituals. There have been times when I've dropped just some of my good habits, and other times when I've dropped them all. Mirroring was often the first to go. Eventually, though, I would reach a state of being disconcerted and dissatisfied in my life, which would lead me back to daily reflection. As soon as I began mirroring again, the first thing I would notice is how insecure, defensive, unmotivated, and uncreative I had been during the time I had neglected this practice.

Living with discipline takes effort, but living without discipline takes even more effort. Even though I am fully aware of this, I still occasionally become lax about mirroring and certain other rituals. Each time, my denial tactics become less effective, and I realize sooner that I would be a lot happier and healthier if I were practicing reflection and other good habits. I try not to be too hard on myself about these times, and to see them as opportunities to appreciate how much better I feel when I'm living consciously and in what I call the "zone of bliss."

goals, however often they may change, helps us to stay motivated on our paths.

On the facing page is a questionnaire that I have used in taking personal inventory. It's a good tool for beginning the mirroring process. You don't have to do this in-depth inventory every day. But you can return to this inventory annually or seasonally. It's a good idea to save your answers so you can look back on them to see how you fared in taking steps toward your goals. Looking over all of the achievements you've made can provide you with a wonderful sense of accomplishment.

The Business of Being questionnaire can be a little bit intimidating. It forces you to become aware of all the realities in your life and the habits, good and bad, that you've been maintaining. But once you have completed it, you will have the first important tool for mirroring and planning the changes you want to make in your life.

You can refer to this questionnaire often, to see how far you've come and to remind you of your goals. I would suggest copying it and putting it with your journal in your meditation space for easy access. But remember, don't be too hard on yourself or just give up if you go through days or periods during which you are not able to live up to all your personal goals and expectations. This questionnaire is meant to help you be conscious of your choices, not to judge yourself.

. . . ON THE WALL

Where you do your mirroring, or inventory, is a matter of personal preference. You can do it at your desk at work, in the bathtub while you're being relaxed through aromatherapy, or in a special place you create for yourself to get away from it all.

Create in your house a space that is your sanctuary. A space to which you go home, where you do your confessions. Where you study the bliss and the crises in your life and create new opportunities instead of blaming the world. When I sit down at my meditation seat at my home in Osceola, Wisconsin, I immediately feel the sacredness of this special spot I've created. I have filled it with things that remind me of the divine, within myself and all things, and I am immediately transported to a place of nurturing—an emotional place that feels like home.

In fact, I treat my entire home as a sacred place, and I recommend this highly. I diffuse aromas I love throughout the house. I have filled it with art, furniture, and objects that inspire comfort and pleasant feelings within me.

❧ EXPLORING AN INSPIRED LIFE

Answer the following questions in as much detail as possible. You will not be sharing this information with anyone, so please be as thorough as possible.

1. ENERGY

 a. How alive do I feel today? How much of my time qualifies as "having fun"?

 b. What do I do to feel young in heart and spirit?

 c. What other things could I do to stay young at heart?

 d. What type of energy do I give to others? Does my energy nourish or deplete others?

 e. Where do I expend most of my life's energy?

2. WORK

 a. Is my work a calling or simply a job? Why?

 b. Do I experience joy in my work?

 c. Do others experience joy as a result of my work?

 d. Am I able to be my true self at work? What part of myself do I "check at the door"?

 e. Do I live my values at work? If yes, how?

 If no, how does this affect other parts of my life?

3. TIME

 a. How do I currently allocate my time? I would create a pie chart of my typical day, using percentages/pie segments to represent the different tasks/obligations/activities, in this way:

 b. Now create a second pie chart of how you would ideally allocate your time during your workday. Include elements you are currently not incorporating but would like to.

4. LEADERSHIP

 a. What does leadership mean to me?

 b. Who has influenced my leadership style?

 c. What have been leadership turning points in my life?

 d. What does power mean to me?

 e. What does empowerment mean to me?

5. SPIRITUAL WELL-BEING

 a. What does spirituality mean to me?

 b. Where do I experience awe in my life?

c. What spiritual fulfillment am I seeking?

d. Where do I go to feed my soul?

e. What does spiritual wellness mean to me?

6. Relationships

in my personal relationships:

a. What does intimacy mean to me?

b. I would describe my most nutritious relationship in this way:

c. Why is this relationship important to me?

d. What areas would I like to enhance within this relationship?

in my work relationships:

a. Do I let others at work really get to know me?

b. With whom do I have the most nutritious relationships at work?

c. What more would I like them to know about me? What creativities, passions, and talents would I like to share?

d. What areas would I like to enhance in my work relationships?

7. Values

To maintain my integrity and direction, I need to clearly define my values. I would complete the following sentences in this way:

a. My most deeply held values are . . .

b. Regarding my role in my community, I believe . . .

c. Regarding my responsibility for the environment, I believe . . .

d. Regarding my relationship to others, I believe . . .

e. I believe success is . . .
   How will I know when I've achieved success as I have defined it?

f. I believe happiness is . . .
   What can I do to experience this daily?

8. Meaning

a. What is my purpose? Why am I here?

b. Do I live true to my purpose in my personal life?

c. Do I live true to my purpose in my professional life?

d. What are some actions I could take to live true to my purpose?

e. Do I need a greater sense of meaning in my life?

f. What will my life's legacy be?

g. How will I pass my legacy on?

I have also adopted the Asian tradition of leaving my shoes, and, symbolically, the stresses of the outside world, at the door. I encourage my guests to do the same, with a sign at the door that reads: "The ritual of removing shoes is welcomed. The purpose is to leave stress and impurities outside and invite joy and peace in. Welcome." Underneath the sign, my guests find a basket full of cozy slippers they can borrow while visiting the special sanctuary I call home.

In our mirroring, wherever we do it, we should develop positive affirmations that can lead us closer to our goals and closer to bliss. We should strive to adopt a habit of looking for the good in everything, even when it is difficult. These affirmations will come out of our analyses of the things in our lives that are working and aren't working. We can use those affirmations to fuel our action and have them work even deeper by contemplating them during our meditation.

Mirroring can be done before meditation or all by itself. Mirroring prior to meditation is useful because it puts us in a contemplative mind-set, a good place to be as we enter the meditative state.

ZONING IN

Meditation is one of the most universal practices in the world. It has been done throughout history by people of all religions and cultures. Every religion has a tradition regarding meditation, so we can feel comfortable meditating regardless of our particular faith.

Still, skeptics may not recognize the great value behind something as passive as sitting still while focusing on one simple thought or affirmation. But the least we all can do, regardless of our initial stance on this practice, is to try it. So many find that meditation is a wonderful source of centering for the mind, body, and spirit. It brings balance to our lives and promotes our growth. People who meditate tend to be calmer, more rational, more hopeful, more creative, more open and receptive to new ideas, and healthier in general. They are often also nicer people to hang out with! This is because meditation is an act through which we strengthen the connection between our mind, body, and spirit and focus all of our systems on our intent. Through slow, steady breath; faith; and directed thought, we gently reacquaint all the sectors of our beings and prepare ourselves to act. It is concentration with surrender. That's the main point of meditation. The idea behind that ritual of sitting still and bringing ourselves close to the alpha state is to summon up from all levels of our being whatever we need

ANY WHICH WAY YOU CAN

There are many different levels of meditation, and many different ways to approach it. There is the sort of meditation in which we sit still and completely clear our minds of all but one thought. And on a much broader scale, there is what I call meditation in action, in which we keep ourselves constantly conscious and in a calm state, so that we are prepared to make intelligent choices about our actions during all of our waking hours. This is a goal to build up to over time.

In between those two ideals, there are many "degrees" of meditation. For example, meditation can be simply taking a leisurely walk in nature, slowing down your breath, and clearing your mind to make room for awareness of all the nature around you. You can meditate sitting or standing, with your eyes closed or open. Gazing at one object without blinking is a form of meditation frequently used for bolstering willpower.

The most important thing about choosing a mode of meditation, though, is to choose the one that works best for you. If you prefer standing with your eyes open while you meditate, don't let anyone tell you that's not the way to do it. Find a comfortable position in a comfortable, nurturing environment—do whatever you have to do so that you can be still and connect with yourself.

to take action, to make real the things we understand we want when we take inventory. We go into the stillness of meditation so that we can transcend into action later.

People have different ideas about what meditation is. There are many who are intimidated because they believe that they have to completely clear their minds. The truth is, we cannot think about absolutely nothing. But, as we meditate, we can reduce the number of channels our minds are accustomed to flipping through. I find meditation to be most effective when I prepare for it by putting myself into a very passive state. To reach this state, I first do some slow breathing exercises. Slowing the breath brings me close to the alpha state, the relaxed stage that precedes sleep. As I discussed earlier, it has been proven that each time we inhale, a new thought enters the mind. Following this train of thought, we see that taking fewer, slower breaths means having fewer thoughts. I find that I have the highest state of focus when I experience the greatest state of relaxation.

There is no prescribed length of time for meditation. I think we should sustain it for as long as we can—whether that's five minutes or an hour. Any amount of time spent meditating provides us with benefits. The longer you stay focused on one object or subject, the closer you get to the state of alpha, a state that is very conducive to healing and self-renewal. That is where self-realization is most likely to occur, especially after you've done contemplation or mirroring.

Once we're calm and breathing slowly, we can meditate. Focus on an affirmation, or an affirming chant. Make that thought the only concern of the mind, and then release it to the universe. (Everything I have wished for in life, I have received after I released the desire in meditation!) Let the mind, body, and spirit coalesce as your continue to breathe slowly and relax the mind. Surrender.

THE LANGUAGE OF MEDITATION: AFFIRMATIONS AND MANTRAS

Words are incredibly powerful. They are the link between thought and action. Expressing an intention out loud or on paper makes it much more real, more doable.

Although meditation is often associated with being in silence, there are words that go along with this practice. They are spoken in two forms—as affirmations of our intent before and/or after meditation, and as mantras during meditation.

PRELUDE TO BLISS

There are yogis and other trained people who can go in and out of meditation very quickly, as if they were turning a light switch on and off. But for most of us, getting calm, still, and focused requires preparation. Here are some steps to consider:

- Create a positive mind-set. Decide that you are going to recognize the positive aspects of your life so that you can strive to keep the good things going, and use the painful experiences of the past as opportunities to make changes for the better.
- Help yourself set your mood by pleasing your senses. Over just a short period of time, you can create a code of stimuli that, through memory response, your brain will come to recognize as nurturing and relaxing. Among those stimuli might be pleasing plant-based aromas and some mood-enhancing music. The idea is to find things that will quickly transport you from the stresses of the outside world to your peaceful, sacred home world.
- Get lost in an idea and surrender yourself to it, once you're ready to meditate. Have faith in that one thought without judging it or trying to come up with another thought.

It is also important to make a slow transition out of meditation.

- Leave enough time in your meditation routine to emerge slowly.
- Come out of your meditation naturally, when possible. Something will usually rouse you, whether it's sitting in the same position for too long, or having a random thought. If, however, you're concerned that you won't come out of your meditative state with enough time to do the other things you need to do, set a timer of some sort—perhaps a diffuser filled with energizing plant-based aromas such as sage or juniper or another of your favorites.
- Consider giving thanks. When I come out of meditation, I go into a state of gratitude, which I recommend. I thank the divinities for the divine experience of meditation, and for all that is in my life.
- Take a moment to make affirmations about your goals before moving on to any other tasks or activities.
- Now comes the meditation in action part: Live up to those affirmations you've made.

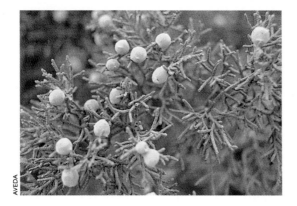

AVEDA

Juniper's pungent aroma may help you keep your meditative focus.

Ylang-ylang's stress-fighting properties may help you ease from a busy day into a peachful meditation.

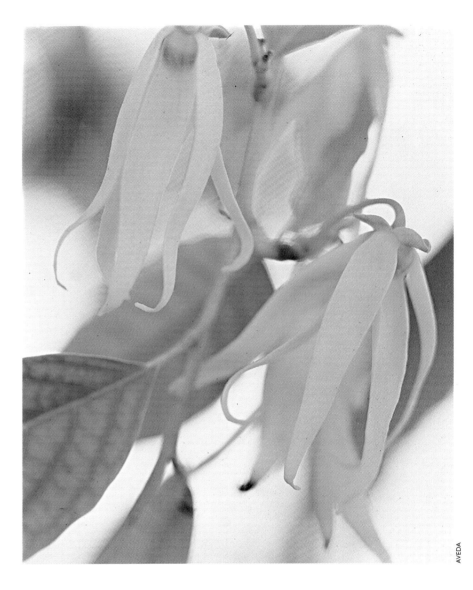

AVEDA

There are no right or wrong affirmations or mantras. Choosing the words for your meditation routine is a very personal matter. Your affirmations will have to do with your personal intent. Your mantra or mantras may also be related to your intent, or they may be given to you by a teacher. Whatever words you choose to utter, make sure they have real meaning to you.

While they are both part of the same process, affirmations and mantras are distinct from each other. Affirmations are statements of what we mean to do and be. If you believe that you are your word, then stating that you are what you intend to be is a simple link to becoming it. The language of affirmations is always positive and focuses on the end result rather than the process. Words like hope, wish, and want don't belong in your affirmations. For example, if your intention is to lose weight, rather than "I will lose weight," or "I hope to lose weight," the affirmation should be: "I *am* losing weight." As you state your affirmations, you should also visualize the end result.

Mantras, put simply, are phrases that help us to become conscious of the divinity within and around us. They can be very simple or very complex strings of words, in our own language or in another. It is important to know the meaning of your mantras. You should always infuse them with positive intent, for mantras are powerful. Their meanings are meant to awaken you to the miraculousness of life, and the powerful, divine life force that makes each of us a sacred entity within a larger sacred community. But, we've all heard of curses and black magic. These are the results of powerful, negative intent. Keep your words and the spirit you put behind them positive.

There is also an aural, sensory component to your mantras. The sound vibrations you create as you chant a mantra are meant to be part of your nurturing sensory experience during meditation. These vibrations also act as conductors for a positive flow of life energy, a recharging of the pranic batteries. You want to breathe deeply before you release your mantra from your lips, and then stretch out the phonetics very slowly so as to prolong the positive meaning and the sensory experience. Put your whole self into it. Hear it. Feel it. Through sense memory response, your brain comes to associate those sound vibrations with their meaning and with pleasant experiences. Over time, just hearing yourself utter your mantras will help to bring you quickly to a meditative state.

SETTING THE MOOD

Meditation should be done at least once a day. If you enjoy it and want to meditate more often, you can practice as long or as often as you like. While we can meditate just about anywhere, the special, comfortable sanctuaries I recommended creating for mirroring are also perfect for meditation. You can aid your passage into a meditative state with some nurturing food for your senses as well. That can include calming sounds, such as recorded music, aromatic candles or incense, comfortable fabrics, and visuals that inspire you. Lots of people create altars for their private sanctuary spaces. They place images of their loved ones and their spiritual coaches, along with symbols of their faith(s) on display so that they'll be reminded of all the nurturing support in their life. If this concept appeals to you, I encourage you to gather special items in a quiet place that you can go to for this healing practice.

FORTY-THREE WAYS TO SAY "I AM"

Mantras are very special phrases, especially when they are given to you by a coach or teacher who knows you well. My teacher, Swami Rama, gave me forty-three mantras, each of which is used for different intentions in meditation. While they're all unique, what these mantras have in common is that they are a path to the divine within and without.

I can't reveal my particular mantras. They're personal. I recommend that you keep your mantras to yourself, too.

There are universal mantras, though, which everyone can share. If you haven't yet been given a mantra by a teacher or developed your own, you can start either with "om" or "so hum." These are both Sanskrit terms that are very commonly used. They may be low on syllables, but they're high on meaning.

"Om," which should be stretched out through a long exhalation and pronounced "a-a-o-o-u-u-m-m-m," means "I am all of that which is divine." "So hum," which can be divided over two breaths, is translated to mean "I am." That may seem terribly simple, but the greater meaning of the statement "I am" is: "I recognize my connection to my individual self and the greater, collective self, and the divinity within everything."

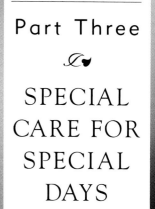

Part Three

SPECIAL
CARE FOR
SPECIAL
DAYS

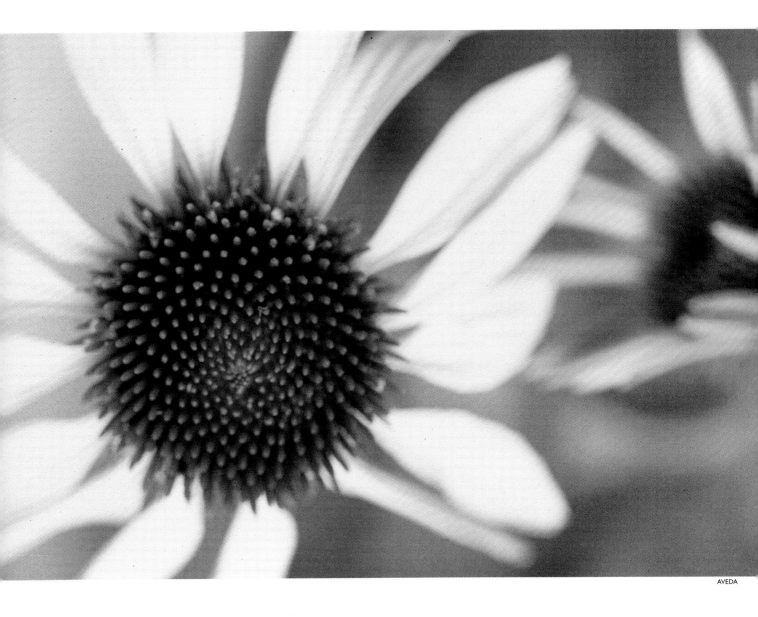

AVEDA

Restoring Balance

Energy Healing

He who smiles rather than rages, is always the stronger.

—JAPANESE PROVERB

T HERE ARE TIMES WHEN ALL OUR ATTEMPTS TO BE healthy fail us. Our daily routines get disrupted for one reason or another. Our lives get hectic, we get run-down, and we become prone to dis-ease, which leads to illness.

No matter how healthy and nurturing our daily practices are, and no matter how diligent we are about them, from time to time, every one of us will likely experience sickness to some degree. Stress or fear or loneliness will find their way into our systems, and our bodies will be affected and react with symptoms. Or, external factors such as exposure to powerful viruses or bacterias will overcome our immunity, and we'll catch a cold, the flu, or a stomach virus. Many of us are also prone to more serious illnesses, such as cancer, hypertension, and heart conditions because of heredity, lifelong stress, harmful lifestyle choices such as smoking, or occupational hazards. We must help our systems fight these intruders and regain their balance.

SICK AND TIRED

Disease often begins on a microscopic, cellular level. Every cell in our body is programmed to protect the body from intruders like bacterias, yeasts, viruses, and free radicals. Different cells have different functions toward guarding the body, which is the biological intelligence of our bodies at work. When disease or emotional distress strikes, some cells become confused and begin to change their activities. The cell's innate intelligence is changed by the intruder. When a healthy cell is invaded by cancer, it is redesigned. It's as if that cell has been signed up by an opposing team and turns against its former teammates. That cancerous cell is now interested in recruiting new members for the cancer team. The consciousness of that cell has gone from renewing consciousness to destructive consciousness. As a result, the body becomes more toxic and stressed, and a perfect breeding ground for more destructive cells.

THE ART OF THE HEAL

Whatever we encounter in terms of disease, we do have the ability to be cured, if not all the way, then to a great degree. Healing is actually second nature to us since the greatest source of healing is within ourselves. Recovery is one of our body's autonomic functions, because of life energy stored within us. This healing energy is present and accessible in all life forms and in every organic particle. It flows through us naturally, as part of the greater life force energy known as *prana* in Sanskrit, *chi* in the Chinese tradition, *ki* in the Japanese culture, and *creative force* among Native Americans.

Stress, the greatest source of illness, blocks the flow of that intelligent energy which directs function. When the flow of life energy in our bodies is blocked, our healing capacities are hampered. Through the intelligence of nature, and our conscious assistance through a change of habits, we can unlock that energy and redirect it to bring renewal and healing to areas that have become dormant and imbalanced.

An open, active mind-body-spirit connection is vital to directing this healing energy. In order to heal we must be positive in our thinking and have faith. It is clear that there is a dualism to our consciousness. There is a consciousness that can destroy, and a consciousness that can renew. In developing a set of nurturing daily habits, we are clearly trying to connect with the consciousness that renews. That renewing consciousness allows for the free flow of life force energy and healing energy. If we look to build and enhance this awareness of the positive energy around us and within us, each day we have an opportunity to promote our personal healing and balance.

We can heal ourselves, and we can be healed by the people and things with whom we have relationships. In order to rely on those people and things when we need them, we must heal them, in turn. The same is true for our relationship with our surroundings. When we contribute to the healing of the Earth and the environment, the Earth and environment pay us back by providing us with a healthier place in which to live and breathe.

There are many symbiotic relationships of which we need to be aware in order to heal ourselves and our world. This is where the quality of our daily nurturing habits becomes vital. They need to be practices that are truly nurturing to ourselves and all that touches us. In addition, our habits need to be practices we love, because love is what heals. When we experience things that arouse feelings of love within us, we are on the road to recovery. Incorporating these healing, renewing activities and thoughts into our daily lives is practicing self-love, which is also self-healing.

WE ARE ALL ONE

Love is one factor in healing. Faith is another big one. All religions address healing in their great books and in their prayer traditions. We have all heard stories about people who prayed for their health when recovery seemed impossible and were subsequently revived. Yet we are always surprised by this. It is always considered a miracle that faith leads to healing.

Another phenomenon that has been noted is when *other* people's prayers seem to promote healing in the ones they love or care about. I recently read a story in Larry Dossey's wonderful book *Be Careful What You Pray For*, about a young man who was dying of AIDS. He had no faith in anything spiritual, but his mother was a very religious woman. She was able to get three hundred people together to pray for her son's recovery. Even though he was thousands of miles away from those who prayed for him—even though he had no idea this group was praying for him—the young man made a miraculous recovery.

THE "NEW" HEALING TRADITIONS

Anyone who labels alternative healing traditions such as homeopathy and herbal medicine "new" could use a history lesson. In recent years there has been a return to less invasive, more natural healing traditions like these, and the only thing that's new about them is scientific documentation that they really work. Many of these practices have actually been used for ages.

When I was a boy growing up in rural Austria, there were apothecaries on every corner of the town. Those apothecaries were stocked predominately with herbal medicines. Modern medicine could be found in the cities, but herbal medicine was what the people in the mountains and the remote places relied upon. My mother was an herbalist in our town. I used a lot of what I learned from her in formulating many of the recipes for AVEDA.

When I traveled to India in the late sixties and early seventies to learn from Swami Rama, I became aware of Ayurveda, the ancient Hindu medical tradition that is being used more and more today in conjunction with so-called orthodox Western medicine. It all made so much sense: Our bodies, minds, and spirits have particular makeups, and when the elements they're influenced by go out of balance, we get sick. We can stay well by knowing our makeups and keeping them in balance.

MEDITATION'S LIFE CHANGING BENEFITS

I also learned firsthand about the power of meditation in healing the body and mind. My wife at the time was stricken with uterine cancer. Swami Rama prescribed specific approaches to meditation. And in a short while, my wife was healed.

I witnessed the effects of meditation in laboratory experiments that were performed on Swami Rama at the University of Minnesota. He could lower his heart rate, alter his brain waves, and decrease his need for air.

Through my meditation in India and at home, it became clear to me that it was important for me to make plant-based products from sustainable resources. That purpose presented itself to me in my stillness. Appropriately, then, while I was in India I met an herbalist named Shivnath Tandof, who was involved in making penicillin in the foothills of the Himalayas. I brought him back with me to start making formulas for AVEDA. Later on, Prakash Purohit—an organic chemist who also has degrees in marketing and finance—joined us from India and helped me found the company incorporating the age-old, healthful, holistic principals I now believe in so strongly.

Many of us believe in a divine universal consciousness. To me, it is obvious that this consciousness exists and is present in all living things on this planet. It is part of nature.

Actually, modern scientists have done research into this phenomenon and have discovered that healing is clearly linked to belief. Through transcendence of belief, an energy is activated. This energy is believed to carry a healing force.

There's actually a scientific explanation for the way in which consciousness can heal. From consciousness, from thought, comes energy. Healing consciousness creates healing energy. Any energy that exists can be managed, directed, and channeled into areas where energy is absent.

It has been documented that directed energy can renew and restore tissues and cells, and even eliminate tumors and disease. It also appears as if healing energy is transferable from one person to another. The Japanese healing tradition of Reiki, which is gaining wider acceptance these days, utilizes touch to direct energy to the regions of the body in which there have been blockages. A Reiki practitioner, through light touch and channeling energy from him- or herself to the patient, can help heal all sorts of ailments from emotional stress to cancer. The Reiki practitioner is really only a facilitator, though. It is the self, through the life force within (the *ki* in Reiki), that is doing the healing.

A GOOD FOOTING

Another powerful Asian healing tradition is reflexology, in which the soles of the feet are studied to understand what's happening in the rest of the body, and massaged as a mode of healing various organs and glands throughout it. Just as the face is a road map for what is happening in the rest of the body, the soles of the feet bear telltale signs of what is occurring in all of our body systems. Calluses, pain, swelling, or irritation in certain areas of the feet may indicate trouble in corresponding organs or glands.

The diagram on the next page indicates the correlation between the areas of the feet and other body parts.

There is a special massage technique to reflexology that we can be use to heal many ailments. We can have reflexology massages done by trained professionals, our partners, and even ourselves. These massages can be done regularly for preventative purposes, or just when we need to heal ourselves. Here's a step-by-step guide.

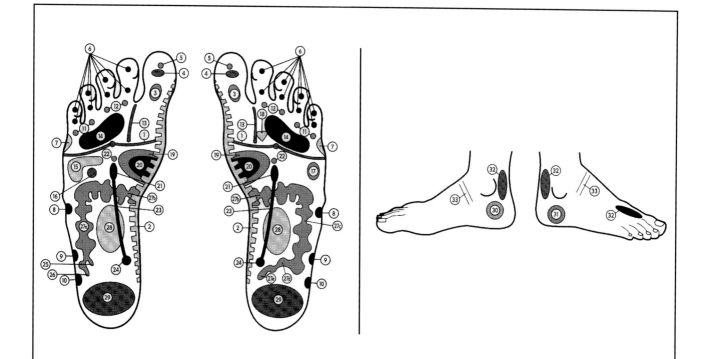

FOOT REFLEXOLOGY POINTS

1. diaphragm

2. spine

3. thyroid, parathyroid and throat

4. pituitary gland

5. treatment benefits

6. sinus ponits

7. shoulder

8. elbow

9. hip

10. knee

11. eyes

12. ears

13. esophagus

14. lungs

15. liver

16. gallbladder

17. spleen

18. heart

19. stomach

20. pancreas

21. kidneys

22. adrenal glands

23. ureter tube

24. bladder

25. ileocaecal valve

26. appendix

27a. ascending colon

27b. transverse colon

27c. descending colon

27d. sigmoid colon

27e. rectum

28. small intestines

29. sciatic nerve

30. uterus/prostate

31. ovaries/testicles

32. lymphatic drainage

33. fallopian tubes/vas deferens

FOOT REFLEXOLOGY MASSAGE

TREATMENT PROCEDURE

Note: All massage manipulations should be a circular friction motion unless otherwise indicated. The reflex points stimulate areas on the same side of the body as the foot being worked on. For example: If you are massaging the lung point on the left foot, you are stimulating the left lung.

With your partner lying faceup, begin the massage by placing your hands under the ankles (left hand to right foot, right hand to left foot). As the client exhales, gently stretch the legs toward you.

Apply product to right foot (you may reapply product during the treatment if needed). Begin the massage on the right foot.

Massage the inside of the right ankle (uterus/prostate point) with the right thumb, simultaneously rotating the ankle with the left hand, which is placed at the base of the toes.

Massage the outside of the ankle (ovary/testicle point) with the left thumb simultaneously rotating the ankle with the right hand, which is placed at the base of the toes.

Massage the diaphragm area with both thumbs using an effleurage motion. As your partner inhales, the thumbs move to meet at the center point for the diaphragm. As your partner exhales, the thumbs move from the center point out. Repeat three times.

Massage the inside arc of the right foot (spinal points) with the right thumb, using an effleurage motion starting at the heel and working toward the big toe. Stop and use a circular friction motion on any tense areas.

Massage the thyroid, parathyroid, and throat points on the right foot with the right thumb.

Massage the pituitary gland and pineal gland points on the right foot (big toe), using the right thumb.

Massage the sinus points on the right foot (second toe to fifth toe) using either thumb.

Massage down the outside of the right foot with the left thumb using an effleurage motion, stopping on the shoulder, elbow, hip, and knee points. Use a circular friction movement on the specific points.

Massage the ear and eye points on the right foot, using either thumb.

Massage down the esophagus area, using either thumb with an effleurage motion. Stop and use a circular friction motion on any tense areas.

Massage the lung area on the right foot, using both thumbs. Be sure to cover the entire lung area.

Massage the liver area (spleen point on the left foot) on the right foot, using the left thumb. Be sure to cover the entire liver area.

Massage the gallbladder point (heart point on the left foot) or the right foot, using the left thumb.

Massage the stomach and pancreas area on the right foot, using both thumbs. Be sure to cover the entire stomach and pancreas area.

Massage the kidney and adrenal gland points on the right foot using the right thumb.

Massage down the ureter tube area, using an effleurage motion with the right thumb. Stop and use a circular friction motion on any tense areas.

Massage the bladder point on the right foot, using the right thumb.

Massage the ileocaecal valve and appendix points on the right foot, using either thumb (right foot only).

RIGHT FOOT: Massage the ascending colon on the right foot, using the left thumb with an effleurage motion. Stop and use a circular friction motion on any tense areas. Massage the trasverse colon on the right foot with the left thumb in the same manner.

LEFT FOOT: Massage the transverse colon on the left foot with the left thumb with an effleurage motion. Stop and use a circular friction motion on any tense areas. Massage the descending colon, sigmoid colon, and rectum on the left foot with the right thumb in the same manner.

Massage the small intestine area on the right foot, using both thumbs. Be sure to cover the entire small intestine area.

Massage the sciatic nerve area on the right heel, using both thumbs. Be sure to cover entire heel.

Massage the uterus/prostate point on the right foot, using the right thumb. Using an effleurage motion toward the heart, massage the inside of the ankle with the right hand to stimulate the lymphatic system.

Massage the ovary/testicle point on the right foot, using the left thumb. Using an effleurage motion toward the heart, massage the outside of the ankle with the left hand to stimulate the lymphatic system.

Massage the top of the right foot with the fingertips of both hands, using an effleurage motion starting in between the toes and working toward the ankle. Be sure to massage the entire top of the foot. This stimulates the lymphatic drainage points.

Massage the fallopian tubes/vas deferens area with the right middle finger, using an effleurage motion from the outside of the ankle to the inside.

Pull each toe gently on both feet to complete the right foot.

Apply product to left foot.

Massage the inside of the left ankle (uterus/prostate point) with the left thumb simultaneously rotating the ankle with the right hand, which is placed at the base of the toes.

Massage the outside of the left ankle (ovary/testicle point) with the right thumb simultaneously rotating the ankle with the left hand which is placed at the base of the toes.

Repeat steps starting with massage of diaphragm area on the left foot.

Note: Use the opposite thumb when massaging the left foot. *For example:* If you use the right thumb to massage a point on the right foot, use the left thumb on the left foot.

Place your hands under the ankles (left hand to right hand, right hand to left foot). As your partner exhales, gently stretch the legs toward you.

HEALING HERBS

TO CLEANSE THE BOWEL AND BLOOD:

- Alfalfa extract contains chlorophyll, which aids in detoxifying the body.

- Aloe vera has a healing and cleansing effect on the digestive tract and aids in forming soft stools.

- Milk thistle aids liver function and enhances bile output to soften stools.

- Herbs that are helpful for constipation include cascara sagrada, goldenseal, rhubarb root, senna leaves, and yerba mate.

- To rebuild the liver and cleanse the bloodstream, use dandelion, milk thistle, red clover, and wild yam.

- Slippery elm is good for inflammation of the colon.

TO EASE STOMACH:

- Alfalfa supplies needed vitamin K and trace minerals.

- Aloe vera is good for heartburn and other gastrointestinal symptoms.

- Anise seeds can help relieve a sour stomach.

- Catnip, chamomile, fennel, fenugreek, goldenseal, papaya, and peppermint are all good for indigestion.

- Ginger is a remedy for nausea.

- Licorice promotes healing of gastric and duodenal ulcers.

TO AID PROSTATE:

- Pygeum and saw palmetto are helpful. European studies suggest pygeum may prevent prostate cancer.

- Buchu, carnivora, echinacea, goldenseal, pau d'arco, and suma have all shown anticancer properties.

- Damiana and licorice root have the ability to balance hormones and glandular function.

- Gravel root, hydrangea, oat straw, parsley root, uva ursi, and yarrow are diuretics that also dissolve sediment.

TO HELP FEMALE ORGANS:

- Damiana enhances sexual desire and pleasure.

- Anise, black cohosh, fennel, licorice, raspberry, sage, sarsaparilla, squawvine, unicorn root, and wild yam root are natural estrogen promoters.

- Gotu kola and dong quai relieve hot flashes, vaginal dryness, and depression.
- Siberian ginseng aids in relieving depression and in the production of estrogen.

TO SUPPORT LIVER:

- Milk thistle contains some of the most potent liver-protecting substances known. It prevents free radical damage by acting as an antioxidant, protecting the liver; it also stimulates the production of new liver cells.
- Burdock root purifies the blood and restores liver and gallbladder function.
- Dandelion root cleanses the bloodstream and liver and increases the production of bile.
- Garlic aids in the treatment of liver disease.

TO CLEANSE KIDNEYS:

- Buchu aids in controlling bladder and kidney problems.
- Cranberries contain substances that acidify the urine, destroy bacteria buildup, and promote healing of the bladder.
- Dandelion root extract aids in excretion of the kidney's waste products and is very beneficial for nephritis.
- Hydrangea and uva ursi are excellent natural diuretics.
- Marshmallow tea helps to cleanse the kidneys.
- Goldenrod tea, juniper berries, marshmallow root, nettle, parsley, red clover, and watermelon seed tea are other herbs that are beneficial for kidney problems.
- Aloe vera juice can be useful in preventing stone formation.
- Ginkgo biloba and goldenseal, taken in extract form, aid circulation to the kidneys and have antiinflammatory properties.

TO BOLSTER HEART AND LUNGS:

- Alfalfa, borage seed, horsetail, nettle, and pau d'arco are rich in minerals necessary for proper regulation of heart rhythm.
- Oat straw, passionflower, valerian root, and skullcap are calming herbs that may help to regulate arrhythmias.
- Butcher's broom, hawthorn berries and leaf, motherwort, and red sage strengthen the heart muscle.
- Cayenne, ginger root, and ginkgo biloba strengthen the heart and are helpful for chest pain.
- Gotu kola, primrose, and rosemary are helpful in managing angina.
- Green tea has antioxidant properties. Ten to twenty cups a day can provide protection against heart disease and many other illnesses.

TO PURIFY LYMPHATIC SYSTEM:

‣ Siberian and panax ginsengs, hawthorn leaf and flower, astragalus, goldenseal, garlic, cayenne, echinacea root, chaparral, and dandelion help to stimulate the lymph glands, promoting lymphatic drainage

TO CHARGE BRAIN:

‣ Ginkgo biloba increases blood flow to the brain.

‣ Anise, blue cohosh, ginseng, and rosemary are other herbs that are helpful for memory.

‣ Huperzine is found in club moss. Used medicinally for centuries in China to treat fever and various neurological disorders, it was also administered to help restore memory in elderly individuals.

‣ Brahmi is renowned for elevating brain functions, increasing concentration, and more finely honing mental focus.

TO BOOST IMMUNE SYSTEM IN GENERAL:

‣ Astragalus boosts the immune system and generates anticancer cells in the body. It is also a powerful antioxidant.

‣ Bayberry, fenugreek, hawthorn, horehound, licorice root, and red clover all enhance the immune response.

‣ Black radish, dandelion, and milk thistle help to cleanse the liver and the bloodstream.

‣ Boxthorn seed, ginseng, suma, and wisteria contain germanium, a trace element that aids immune function and has anticancer properties.

‣ Echinacea boosts the immune system and enhances lymphatic function.

‣ Goldenseal strengthens the immune system, cleanses the body, and has antibacterial properties.

‣ Picorrhiza, an Indian herb used in Ayurvedic medicine, is a powerful immunostimulant that boosts all aspects of the immune system.

‣ Ligustrum (Chinese *nu zhen zi*) increases bone marrow production of lymphocytes as well as their maturation into T-cells.

SPECIAL TREATMENT

When we're sick we can also restore our body's balance by amplifying those nurturing rituals that have the most gentle healing properties. If we increase the number and frequency of massages when we're not well, we increase the flow of healing energy and help the body rid itself of infection and toxins. (See the Reflexology chart.) At these times we should also drink more teas with antiseptic and cleansing herbs and roots, like ginger, licorice, basil, and peppermint.

When I get a cold, I keep with me a huge thermos filled with warm water, lemon, and ginger, and I drink it all day. This helps me to flush out the infection while cleansing my body and replenishing its moisture.

When we're not feeling well, sometimes it's just a little extra TLC— tender loving care—like this that we need to give ourselves. Do the things that bring you comfort, and do them more than usual. Beyond that, use common sense and see your doctor.

RELAXING RETREATS

When we follow a set of nurturing practices on a daily basis, we continually help our bodies to rid themselves of stressors of all sorts. But in spite of such vigilant daily maintenance, even if we have the most tranquil, peaceful lives, some stress manages to get through our defenses. That stress accumulates, and so from time to time we need to do things that are a little bit more radical in their ability to remove stress and toxins.

A very effective method is a retreat of some sort that takes us away from our regular environment to a more placid place where we can contemplate and detoxify. Detoxification can refer to the elimination of anything and everything from emotional stress to excess sodium in the diet to alcohol in the system. For some people, a relaxing weekend away in the country will have restorative effects. This is a good seasonal or occasional ritual to uphold in your life if it works for you. Try different settings and periods away from your daily routine to find places and times that are most beneficial to your rejuvenation.

In addition, or instead, we can do serious inner cleansing in a remote place where we can really be alone with ourselves for ten days. This includes physical, mental, and spiritual cleansing, through a meager diet, silence, and journal writing. I like to do this once or twice a year, in the spring and the fall, usually in the Himalayas in India.

A lot of people associate cleansing with fasting. Some do fast for five or ten days. I have done this, but I find it more helpful to subsist on liquids, purees, and thin soups for five days at a time. This incites a less harsh change on the body.

The combination of a cleansing, very light diet with silence, and intense journal writing has a very profound effect on all sectors of the being. There is no greater mirror to stand before than the one we encounter during cleansing, when we are far away from our usual distractions and the other details of life that keep us from being totally conscious.

A new, heightened level of consciousness is achieved in these cleansing periods. We have bold revelations about our pasts and about our goals. There are moments during a cleansing period that are very difficult. We are presented with pain that we need in order to grow, but without the usual buffers in our lives. When we emerge from a cleansing and silence period, there is often a great sense of growth and accomplishment.

GRADUALLY AND THEN SUDDENLY

Each day of a five-day cleansing period is different, in terms of diet. Whether we choose to cleanse for five days, more, or fewer, it is important to work into it gradually. Don't just stop eating, or switch to a diet of only lentil broth, without easing into it.

You need to get ready for a cleansing a couple of days before. Start writing things down. Make lists of things you do and don't like about your life. Maybe redo the inventory questionnaire I included in the "Reflections" section. This will help you get ready to be focused on examining your inventory more intensely, to really remove toxins from the mind.

Begin cleansing by eating some vegetable purees. Later in this chapter, you'll find some recipes I use for purees of chickpeas, lentils, and vegetables combined with cleansing herbs and spices such as pepper, licorice, ginger, basil, peppermint, and lemon. It is good to drink infusions with these ingredients throughout the cleansing to help the body get rid of internal toxins.

The purees can be made easily in a blender or food processor. As the cleansing continues, from the third day on, the purees should get thinner until they are brothlike on the last day. After the cleansing it's important to add food back into our diets gradually, too, giving our systems a couple of days to readjust to regular quantities of food.

Keep writing—and not talking—throughout the cleansing ritual. Purge

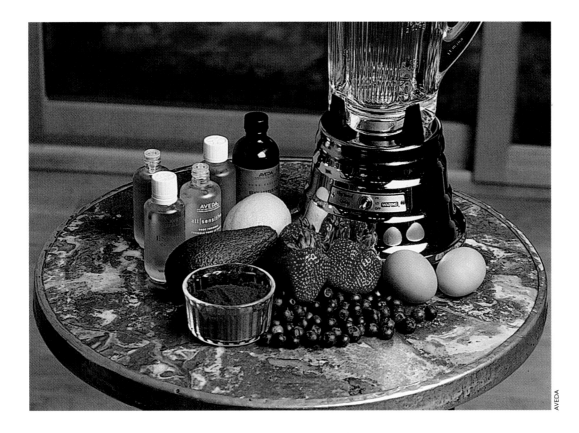

AVEDA

your mind of thoughts, even those that are difficult to face. The sooner we face these demons, the sooner we learn from them and the sooner they stop plaguing us. Remember, what you resist persists.

After the fourth day of cleansing, begin performing enemas on yourself, to encourage elimination of toxins. On the fifth day, take an ounce of castor oil to clean the digestive and elimination systems. (It's a good idea to stay home, or somewhere near a bathroom, that day.)

Our physical exercise during these days of inner cleansing should be limited to gentle yoga and other slow movement traditions, like tai chi. We need to preserve our energy for the arduous task of observing and cleansing the self.

Following are some more specific instructions and recipes to use during your period of inner cleansing.

Cleansing concoctions for the skin and digestive system can be whipped up with a blender, using common foods, spices, and essential oils.

Cleansing Eating

I use the following recipes from *Healthy Healing* by Linda Rector Page when I am doing a cleansing retreat, and I recommend them if you'd like to deeply purify your system. You will need a juicer or blender to create most of these broths and drinks.

FOR ENERGY. HIGH IN MINERALS AND ELECTROLYTES

✁ *Potassium Broth*

Cover the following with water:

    4 carrots
    2 potatoes
    1 onion
    3 celery stalks
    ½ bunch parsley
    ½ head of lettuce
    ½ bunch of broccoli

Simmer 30 minutes. Strain and discard solids.

Add 2 teaspoons of Bragg's Liquid Aminos, a high protein, soy-flavored condiment that can be purchased in most health food stores, or 1 teaspoon of miso. Keep stored in refrigerator.

MACROBIOTIC CLEANSING SOUP

✁ *Rice Purifying Soup*

Toast in a large pan until aromatic (about 5 minutes) the following:

    ⅔ cup lentils
    ⅔ cup split peas
    ⅔ cup brown rice

Add and cook over low heat for 1 hour, stirring occasionally:

    2 cloves minced garlic
    1 onion, chopped
    3 cups water
    3 cups onion or veggie broth
    1 carrot, chopped
    1 stalk celery, chopped
    1 teaspoon cayenne pepper
    ½ teaspoon ginger powder

CLEANSING DRINK WITH BLADDER FLUSHING ACTIVITY

✁ *Purifying Daikon and Scallion Broth*

Heat gently together for five minutes:

    4 cups vegetable broth
    1 six-inch piece daikon radish peeled and cut into matchstick-sized pieces
    2 scallions with tops

Stir in 1 tablespoon tamari, or 1 tablespoon Bragg's Liquid Aminos

1 tablespoon freshly chopped cilantro

a pinch of pepper

A THERAPEUTIC BROTH WITH ANTIBIOTIC PROPERTIES
TO REDUCE AND RELIEVE MUCUS CONGESTION

✺ *Onion/Garlic Broth*

Sauté 1 onion and 4 cloves garlic in $\frac{1}{2}$ teaspoon sesame oil until very soft. Then whirl in the blender with a little vegetable broth. Take in small sips.

BROTH FOR COLD

✺ *Cold Defense Cleanser*

$1\frac{1}{2}$ cups water

1 teaspoon garlic powder

1 teaspoon ground ginger

1 tablespoon lemon juice

1 tablespoon honey

$\frac{1}{2}$ teaspoon cayenne

3 tablespoons brandy

KIDNEY CLEANSER AND DIURETIC DRINK

✺ *Kidney Flush*

4 carrots

4 beets with tops

4 celery stalks with leaves

1 cucumber with skin

8 to 10 spinach leaves

1 teaspoon Bragg's Liquid Aminos (optional)

STOMACH/DIGESTIVE CLEANSER

Juice of $\frac{1}{2}$ cucumber with skin

2 tablespoons apple cider vinegar

8 ounces water

CARROT JUICE PLUS

Juice of 4 carrots
Juice of ½ cucumber
Juice of 2 stalks of celery with leaves
1 tablespoon chopped dry dulse

HIGH PROTEIN JUICE THAT IS GOOD FOR ENDING A FAST

✖ Sprout Cocktail

Juice of 3 cored apples with skin
1 tub alfalfa sprouts
3 to 4 sprigs fresh mint

BLOOD PURIFYING AND IRON ENRICHING DRINK

✖ Blood Builder

Juice of 2 bunches of grapes, or 2 cups grape juice
Juice of 6 oranges, or 2 cups orange juice
Juice of 8 peeled lemons, or 1 cup lemon juice
2 cups water
¼ cup honey

ENZYME ACTIVATOR WITH GINGER TO BREAK UP EXCESS STOMACH ACIDS

✖ Good Digestion Punch

Juice of 1 papaya, peeled and seeded
Juice of 1 pineapple, skinned and cored, or 1 to 2 oranges, peeled
Sliced fresh ginger, or 1 teaspoon cardamom powder

TEA: COMBINATION FOR BLOOD CLEANSING

Red clover	Sage	Horsetail
Hawthorn	Alfalfa	Gotu kola
Pau d'arco	Milk thistle seed	Lemongrass
Nettle	Echinacea	

TEA: COMBINATION FOR MUCUS CLEANSING

Mullein	Pleurisy root	Fennel seed
Comfrey	Rosehips	Ginger
Ephedra	Calendula	Peppermint
Marshmallow	Boneset	

TEA: COMBINATION FOR BOWEL CLEANSING

Senna leaf	Peppermint	Calendula
Papaya leaf	Lemon balm	Hibiscus
Fennel seed	Parsley leaf	Ginger root

TEA: COMBINATION FOR BLADDER AND KIDNEY FLUSHING

Uva ursi
Ginger root
Juniper berries
Parsley leaf

TEA: COMBINATION FOR FATIGUE

2 parts gotu kola
2 parts peppermint
2 parts red clover
1 part clove

PRESCRIPTIONS FOR HEALING

Here are some healing combinations of essential oils to use during massage to help heal the following ailments:

Cold Sores

On cold sores I use straight oils and I apply them repeatedly with a Q-tip. If done every half hour, the cold sore will be gone the next day. I have frequently gotten cold sores since I was a child. I put on any of these oils: peppermint, menthol, thyme, coriander, rose, chamomile, wintergreen, lavender. These are appropriate treatments for cold sores that are outside of the mouth only. Do not apply these oils inside the mouth.

Swollen Eyes

Cut a half slice of potato and apply it directly to the swollen area. Within twenty minutes the swelling should be gone. A freshly cut cucumber also works, but I have not found it as effective as a potato.

Dry, Cracked Skin

Castor oil, jojoba, vitamin E, primrose, borage, avocado, Brazilian nut, and olive oil are all good bases for extremely dry skin. Mix all in equal portions and you'll have a unique combination base to which you can then add essential oils.

Hair and Scalp

Alopecia is hair loss in which the hair usually comes back. Nobody knows exactly what causes it; it can be brought on by anything from stress to hormone changes. To treat it or any less-severe scalp conditions like dandruff, here are some oils to put into a massage base of jojoba: borage or evening primrose, vitamin E, American sage, cedar, rosemary, lavender, rose, or patchouli. Add five drops each in one ounce of base and use daily with acupressure scalp massage.

Colds and Chest Coughs

To treat a cold, drink lots of green tea and echinacea. Massage into the chest the following oils, using a base of jojoba or another of your choice: ginger, cinnamon, vanilla, peppermint, sage, cedar, camphor, eucalyptus, pine, pepper, marjoram, rosemary, and wintergreen.

Fever

Use the same base formula and add rosemary, lemongrass, lemon, lime, sage, cedar, pine, fir needle, wintergreen, camphor, or cinnamon essential oils. Vanilla can be added to each one for a relaxing and calming effect. The essential oil should be about 5 percent of the mix. The resulting oil should be kneaded into the entire body with a quick rubbing motion. Keep your body warm so that you begin to sweat. You can apply a little on your nostrils to help breathing through a stuffed nose. This will bring down your fever, provoke sweating, and make you feel more comfortable.

Anxiety

To soothe anxiety, rub on or inhale aroma of rose, olibanum, jasmine, or neroli.

Depression

To fight depression, use Saint-John's-wort, green tea, rose, jasmine, neroli, ylang-ylang, chamomile, and Roman or German chamomile.

Jet Lag

To fend off weariness, apply a bit of any of the following oils (diluted into a base) onto your nostrils or on a handkerchief that you touch to your nose frequently: rose, jasmine, mandarin, lime bergaruot, or lemongrass. The essential oil should be 5 percent of the mix.

Refreshing Morning Bath

Add rosemary, petitgrain, bergamot, eucalyptus, and peppermint to bathwater.

Cooling Bath

In the summertime add peppermint, eucalyptus, camphor, sage, cedar, or pine to your bath.

Fatigue

Add thyme, rosemary, and peppermint to your bathwater to soothe fatigue.

Overworked, Painful Muscles

Use any of these oils: lavender, marjoram, rosemary, peppermint, wintergreen, or thyme. Dilute in base. Massage onto your body before bathing

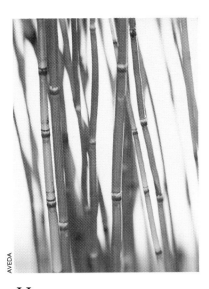

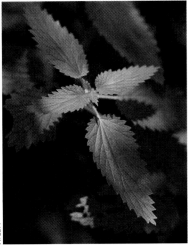

Horsetail and nettle are both stomach soothing remedies.

and continue to rub on the sore area while in the bath. Reapply this essential oil to sore area after your bath and then sleep or rest.

Relaxation and Sleep

Any calming essential oil you love to smell will do the trick.

Baby Massage

Use one drop of chamomile, rose, or neroli in any of the recommended bases, but use one drop each only—never more.

High Blood Pressure

Rose, chamomile, any of the German vanillas, cinnamon, lavender, geranium, neroli, or jasmine. Carry a small bottle with you and apply to nostrils for inhalation through the day. Go on a high protein diet where carbohydrate is secondary to protein with every meal taken. Avoid extra salt and only eat good fats. Walk a lot. Check your blood pressure monthly. Drink lots of green tea. Check with your doctor.

Bronchitis

Essential oils are a good aid in treating bronchitis and other light infections of the lungs through the inhalation of therapy oils like bergamot, eucalyptus, lavender, rosemary, and marjoram. Inhaled, these will assist in easier breathing.

Bruises

Fennel or lavender can be used to heal bruises, or a good homeopathic might be anica and anica ointments. Lavender green ointments are also very useful.

Chemotherapy

Before going to a chemotherapy treatment, mix your favorite essential oil with a massage oil base and apply it directly to your nostrils. This will help prevent nausea.

Pain Killers

Peppermint, camphor, eucalyptus, thyme, rose, sage, cedar, pine, ginger, wintergreen, and rosemary all help reduce the effects of pain when massaged into a sore spot or added to a hot bath.

Low Blood Pressure

Cinnamon, clove, coriander, black pepper, cayenne pepper, American sage, ginger, thyme, and peppermint are all essential oils that will help regulate low blood pressure.

Cellulite

To reduce cellulite, massage trouble spot with a base oil mixed with coriander, thyme, margarine, wintergreen, peppermint, eucalyptus, carrot, or angelica.

Eczema

To treat this skin disorder, apply an equal amount of vitamin E, wheat germ oil, and borage, and add three drops of chamomile, rose, melissa, lavender, geranium, or neroli.

Athlete's Foot

Wintergreen Chinese—if a base of oil or gel of fresh aloe vera is not available, you can use witch hazel, which can be purchased at a pharmacy. Borage oil, jojoba, or grape seed oil also work well. Three drops of wintergreen, three drops marjoram, eucalyptus, geranium, thyme, sage, cedar, peppermint, tea tree, lemon, orange, or mandarin oil. Massage into feet and leave on overnight. In extreme cases, put on cotton stockings and sleep in them. This should take care of it with one treatment; if it returns, repeat the treatment.

Sunburn

For heat rash, use aloe vera gel, lavender water, rose water, chamomile water, or rosemary water. If waters are difficult to make because essential oils don't mix well with water, AVEDA has a process that dissolves essential oils into water. If you can't get those waters, mix these oils with jojoba. Jojoba itself is soothing and healing to a burn. You should apply it in a low dosage of about two drops.

HEALING THE MACROCOSM—THE EARTH

We can allow the healing process to be a self-centered endeavor only up to a point. We must focus on the microcosms of ourselves in order to heal, but we must also consider the health of the macrocosm, the Earth on which we live and depend for our survival. When the Earth and its environment are sick, we are likely to be sick as well.

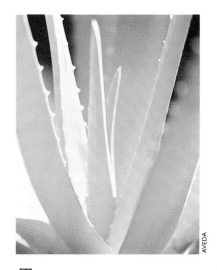

The aloe vera plant produces a gel that helps sunburn and athlete's foot.

Forests are being cut down for the sake of industry, farming, mining, and real estate, depleting the Earth of the plants and trees that heal it. We lose 40 to 50 million acres of forest per year. Virgin forests are becoming extinct, costing us the opportunity to hold on to the original intelligence of plants, which can't be replicated. Only 5 percent of virgin territories remain in the United States. And 90 percent of the species in those forests have never been studied. Those forests are libraries filled with biological information that is being destroyed and cannot be replicated. Pesticides are destroying our food as well as the soil in which our food grows and the water supply. One billion pounds of active ingredients in pesticides are used each year in the United States. It has been projected by some scientists that in ten years, we will all need to cover ourselves before leaving our homes to protect ourselves from environmental protrusions. As it is, many of us are already making sure we never leave home without facial protection, in the form of makeup and sun screens with sun protection factors (SPFs). In ten years, if the environmental pollution increases at the rate it has, we won't be able even to think of going out without something on our skin.

If we stopped all the major sources of harm to the environment today, it would probably take seven generations for the planet to be healthy again. If we keep going the way we are, who knows how long healing will take.

We all need to accept the grand task of healing the Earth, in whatever small ways we each can. Here are some things we can all do:

‣ Buy high-quality products so that they don't need to be replaced often. This will contribute to lowering the pollution that comes from manufacturing.

‣ Buy refrigerators, air conditioners, and other appliances that don't use Freon. Freon destroys ozone, which shields us from the sun. Without ozone, the sun can kill organic life and cause skin cancer. Appliances that don't use Freon may cost a bit more, but who can place a price on a future for our Earth and environment?

‣ Drive a car that has low emissions.

‣ Support organic farming. You'll be healing the small body—your own—and the large body—the Earth.

‣ Stop using products in aerosol cans.

‣ Read up on the companies you patronize. Avoid buying things from companies that are known to pollute.

» Support the companies that are making a difference by reducing pollution and encouraging recycling.

» Educate your kids about the importance of preserving the Earth and the environment. Share with them the enjoyment of nature so they'll have a high appreciation for it. This way, we can have some hope for the future.

» Vote for local and national politicians who make the environment a part of their social agenda.

In the resources section at the end of this book, you'll find information on organizations that are involved in activism and environmentalism. Everyone should align themselves with one or more of these groups—everyone who wants there to be an Earth for future generations to live on, that is.

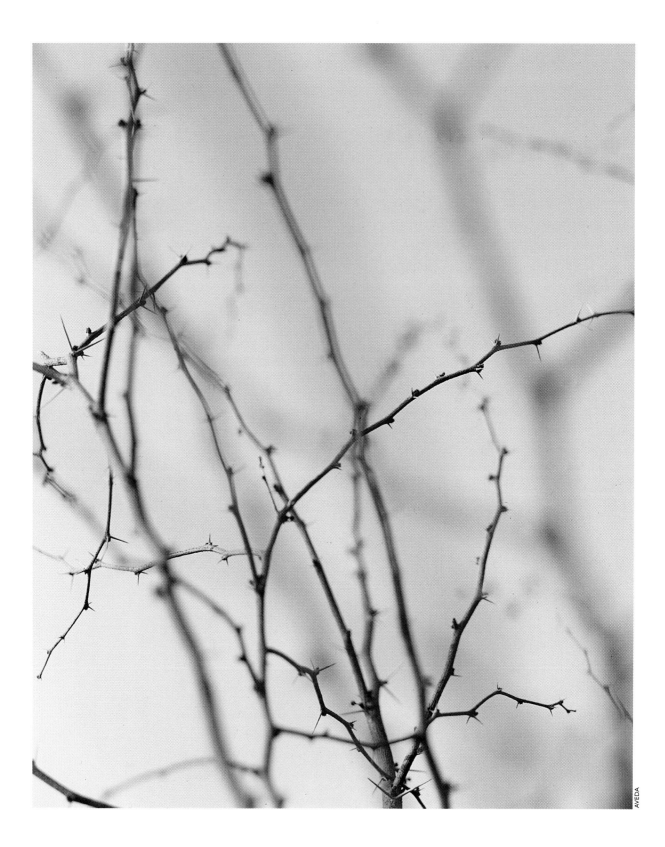

AVEDA

Seasonal Beauty and Celebration

Health and Beauty Through the Seasons

Your self-existence is unchangeable, but your form is subject to change; the whole process of life teaches you that life is nothing but a series of changes. Beneath all these changes lies something that never changes. Grieve not, be aware of both.

—SWAMI RAMA

THE CHANGE OF SEASONS IS ONE OF THE MOST REMARKABLE occurrences in nature. The climate shifts from one extreme to another, and then back again, in an ongoing cycle. The environment you live in transforms so that it seems almost like a completely different place.

The Earth and atmosphere aren't the only things affected by the change of season. Humans are affected, too. We undergo physical, emotional, and spiritual changes as we move from one time of year to another. We make obvious changes in our wardrobes and our activities outdoors. We don't go swimming outdoors in the winter, and we don't wear down-filled parkas in the summer.

We need to make comparable adjustments in our other daily habits, according to the seasons. There are subtle changes that take place in the world around us, which affect every aspect of our beings. There are different intensities and amounts of sunlight, which can affect our need for sun protection and influence our moods. Certain holidays and seasonal customs can affect our spirits. What's more, the changes in weather conditions have a bearing on us, externally and internally. Fluctuations in moisture and temperature manifest changes in the condition of our skin and hair. And being able to spend more or less time in nature can impact emotions.

The seasons affect everyone differently. We each have our favorite and least favorite seasons, for various emotional and physical reasons. Ayurveda teaches us that our doshas, or elemental makeups, dictate which seasons we naturally thrive in and which we might find more difficult. People with a dominant pitta, or fire element, will find the heat of the summer difficult to bear, while people with dominant vata, or air element, will find the cold of the winter uncomfortable. People with a dominant kapha, or earth element, tend to be intolerant of cold, wet weather. Refer to Chapter 3 for a guide to discovering your own dominant doshas and learning in which seasons it's best for you to undertake certain activities and eat certain foods.

But regardless of our individual constitutions, we all need to make certain adjustments and take certain precautions as each quarter approaches. Following are some of the things to consider for each of the four seasons.

WINTER

The winter is fallow, in terms of growing things in the earth, participating in social activities, and for many people, feeling emotions. It's a time of cooler temperatures and, with the exception of snowy or rainy days, dryer air. We need to take all of these things into account as we go into winter, and adjust our rituals concerning our skin and hair.

▸ Drink more water. It's important for hydrating your skin as well as your internal organs. Carry around a bottle of purified water with you for convenience.

▸ Mist your skin frequently with a rose water–based toner to help to keep your skin moist and also refresh your senses.

▸ Moisturize your skin and your hair more frequently. Keep handy all day a small amount of moisturizer, for your face and body, and leave-in conditioner for your hair. Moisturizing foundations are another good source of protection from the dry air.

▸ Don't forget your sunblock. The fact that it's not beach weather does not reduce the harmful effects of too much exposure to direct sunlight. And stay out of the sun or wear a hat during the peak hours of 11 A.M. to 2 P.M.

▶ Use essential oils that have yang, or warming properties, such as cinnamon, vanilla, patchouli, marjoram, clove, myrrh, olibanum, ginger, jasmine and cardamom. You can add these to base oils for self-massage and partner massage to warm you up during the winter months. They can also make a warming bath even warmer.

Winter is a time of hibernation for certain mammals, and for humans, the equivalent is a lowered rate of outdoor and physical activity, and a slower metabolism. These influence our weight. We can counterbalance these influences with special rituals concerning our diet and exercise.

▶ According to Ayurvedic medicine, it is important to consume more protein in the colder weather to sustain your energy.

▶ The holiday season often presents us with lots of rich foods and sweets at every social gathering. It takes willpower to resist these things, and you shouldn't give up on your positive eating habits altogether if you indulge here and there. It is also helpful to make sure that you eat regular, balanced meals so that you're not too hungry at those cocktail parties and office gatherings, and you'll be less apt to grab anything and make excuses like, "Well, I've got to eat *something.*"

▶ It's okay to gain a little weight in the winter. It's natural for your body to insulate itself against the lower temperatures. However, most of us don't want to gain more than a couple of pounds or ounces, and we can control that by exercising more at the gym, or by participating in winter sports such as skiing. If you don't have access to a gym, it's a good idea to buy some home equipment for aerobic, cardiovascular exercise.

We are also more prone to illness in the winter, when the flu and colds are prevalent.

▶ Get a flu shot at the beginning of the season. I have been getting them for the past few years, and I never get sick in the winter anymore.

▶ If you do get sick, drink lots of warm water with lemon, garlic, and ginger for warming and cleansing.

▶ Keep essential oils that you love in your environment and in your pocket for their antibacterial properties.

Emotionally, the traditional winter holidays—including Christmas, Hanukkah, Kwanzaa, and New Year's—can be a time of exuberance or a

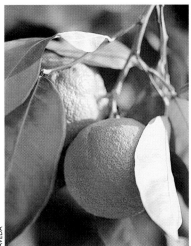

The sun that brings the orange into its ripe glory can rob our hair and skin of moisture. Be sure to protect yours with antioxidents in the warm months.

time of sadness, depending on our own sense memories relating to these times in our lives, as well as our Ayurvedic doshas. We can tailor our meditation and prayer practices, as well as our social interaction, to accommodate those feelings.

▸ Since many people will be making holiday plans, thinking ahead is especially important at this time of year if you want to interact with friends and family and be included in celebrations.

▸ Fight the inclination to stay inside all the time. Get out, even though it's cold. Bundle up and take a walk. Run through the snow. Build a snowman.

SPRING

Spring is a time of change. After a long winter, we open the windows and we let the sun and the fresh air come in to our homes and our hearts. It's a time of cleansing and ridding our selves and our spaces of all that accumulated during the cold weather. Spring cleaning is important in every aspect of our lives.

▸ Our bodies may have gained weight over the winter. Since the temperature is warmer, we can get more exercise outdoors to help shed those extra pounds we might have accumulated. Start walking more and driving less. Dust your bicycle off and use it to do errands as well as to take leisurely rides.

▸ In addition to fat, toxins and emotional stress are also likely to have accumulated in our systems during the colder months. This makes spring a good time to do a mind/body cleansing for five or ten days, with a special diet and lots of personal mirroring and inventory. Refer to the previous chapter where I discuss ways to approach these periods of inner cleansing.

▸ Our skin can use a little extra cleaning after all the extra moisturizer we stocked our pores with in the winter. A facial at a spa is a good way to cleanse the face. You can use cleansing masques at home, too.

▸ It remains important to moisturize, especially since you're likely to be out in the fresh (drying) air more often.

▸ Since you'll probably spend more time outdoors than you did in the winter, pay extra attention to keeping your skin protected from the sun. Wear hats, sunblock, or foundation with SPFs.

SUMMER

Most of us grew up having the summers free. Summer recess from school may not be a part of adult life, unless you're a teacher or academic. But this season is still a great time for vacationing and relaxing, partly because it is good to keep activity levels low during the extremely warm weather.

While summer can inspire a carefree state of mind, it is also a time when we must take extra care to protect ourselves from the elements. The heat can cause us to become dehydrated, internally and externally.

> Make sure you drink more than the usual eight eight-ounce glasses of water over the course of the day, for your skin and your internal organs. Keep a bottle of purified water with you at all times.

> Consume foods and juices with potassium, such as bananas and orange juice, to help keep you from getting dehydrated or suffering from heat prostration.

> Drink lots of teas made with herbs that have yin or cooling properties, such as peppermint, sage, eucalyptus, and lemongrass. During the summer, you can even grow these herbs in your own garden.

> Moisturize your skin, even though perspiration will make your skin a bit more moist than in other seasons. If you have oily skin, you might want to use more water-based rather than oil-based emulsions in your moisturizer, sunblock, or foundation, particularly at this time of year.

> Protect yourself from the sun's harmful rays; it's never more important than during the summer. The sun's rays are more direct and intense. And we spend more time outdoors. Take extra care to cover yourself up, especially during the peak sun hours of 11 A.M. to 2 P.M. Wear hats and use sunblock or foundation with SPFs. The days of sun worshiping are over.

> Protect your hair from the sun, too. AVEDA makes products that coat the hair with silicon and a protein found in Brazil nuts to counteract the heat and sun. You may want to consider using those or other similar products.

> Protect yourself from bugs and ticks, too, if you spend time in nature. But don't use bug sprays that are harmful to yourself or the environment. Try AVEDA's repellent called Attracts Humans, Not Insects, which is made from essential oils. It smells nice—to people only.

Summer barbecues may be appetizing, but too much food in summer can be a bad thing because our bodies and metabolisms are slowed down by the heat.

》 Eat smaller meals more frequently to sustain energy throughout the day.

》 Avoid heavy foods that put stress on the digestive system.

》 Consume more fruits and vegetables, which move through your system more quickly and easily.

Because the weather is more extreme and can affect your energy level, summer is a good time to take a vacation from work, either in a big block, or in several long weekends.

FALL

Things cool off in autumn, and it's time to get back down to business. Our vacation/relaxation mode of summer gives way to more time spent at work. Leaves fall; the air cools and gets dryer. It's a transition into the fallow winter months and a time to prepare for that extreme.

As the climate gets cooler and dryer, it's time to start hydrating more.

》 Drink lots of water, and keep plenty on hand.

》 Begin moisturizing your skin more. If you have oily skin, the fall and winter are the times when your skin will be more receptive to oil-based moisturizers.

In many other ways, fall is similar to winter. You can refer to the precautions and recommendations above for the colder weather.

Being that the fall is the end of the calendar year, it is a great time to take inventory and set new goals for the new year.

》 If you plan to do inner cleansing twice a year, the fall is a good time for one of those periods, particularly for doing inventory on your mind and your soul. It's a good time to empty yourself of the stresses and toxins of the year past, to make room in our minds and bodies for what the new year has to offer. For this reason, I like to go to India for my retreats in the fall. The weather there is also mild during the northern hemisphere's winter.

》 Thanksgiving is perfectly placed in this season. At the close of the year, as we take stock of the previous months, it's a good time to show gratitude for all that is good in our lives. It will make you feel just as good to give thanks as it will for people to receive it.

Days of Celebration, Nights of Magic

We should treat all of our days as if they were special. Regardless of the date, we must welcome the new opportunities and challenges each sunrise delivers, and nurture all our senses continually. But there are some days that are extraspecial, many of which inspire celebration. These occasions that beg for distinct rituals—special mind and body preparations. Birthdays, weddings, anniversaries, holidays, rites of passage, promotions, vacations, family reunions, new births, and even deaths all provide moments that feel different from our ordinary ones.

Our cultures already furnish an array of customs for these occasions, such as particular foods, clothes, prayers, music, gifts, and dancing. These customs definitely help to set our special occasions apart from the average day. So why would we need more new customs? Because it's up to us to carry further into our personal experience the uniqueness of those times. They will have greater resonance if we design a set of *personal* habits to help us rejoice fully, with mind, body, and spirit—a set of habits that varies even from the new daily routines we've just established.

We can also designate new special occasions for ourselves. The ones we already have are great, but why not get creative and establish a time to commemorate whatever you like, once a year, once a season, once a month? Perhaps a seasonal or monthly "me" day, when you don't do anything for anyone but yourself and you escape from even those you love very dearly. Or a weekly couple of days, when you and your partner make time for each other only, to do the things you love together. I have added Earth Day to my roster of special days. I commemorate it by participating in environmental activism in some way, and by having a party at my house where I serve only organic foods and inform those friends who have very little awareness about the importance of organic farming and other environmental issues. I also find annual or semiannual cleansing periods of five to ten days to be very momentous times of self-discovery. I have special nurturing habits for those periods, many of which are simply amplified versions of my daily ones.

Just as there are habits that can nurture us on a daily basis, there are those that should be reserved for occasional use because

- they are broader approaches to some of our daily rituals, such as setting goals for an entire year rather than just an afternoon or a week
- some practices are too expensive to splurge for every day—like professional body work or skin treatments at a spa

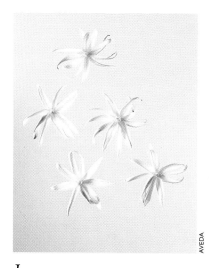

AVEDA

*J*asmine flowers are festive in their beauty and the scent they create can help you commemorate and relive your special occasions—instantly.

› there are some practices that are too extreme to engage in very often—like fasting and observing long periods of silence

In this chapter, I'll discuss some of those rituals that are not a part of our everyday lives, but that can help to mark our time here and make our existences as a whole much richer. Some of them will be for personal, private practice. Others will be for sharing. Get ready to celebrate!

MEMBERS OF THE WEDDING

Some practices that start off as private can later be shared as part of a celebration. It's a way to put a very personal stamp on a momentous occasion, like a wedding. I have a great example to share with you, which comes from my daughter Nicole's wedding, but which originated with her birth.

When Nicole was born, I gave her mother essential oils to inhale during the contractions and the delivery to help ease the pain naturally. I stood by her with a vial of the most fragrant citrus, spice, and floral essences, a combination I liked so much I included it in the AVEDA product line. It's called Valencia and is used in candles and room sprays. That fragrance has always reminded me of the special day my Nicole was born, and has, in my mind, been *her* scent.

Years later, that special ritual I created for her birth gave birth to another one. When it was time for Nicole to be married, I brought the Valencia scent into the celebration for everyone to enjoy. Valencia was everywhere— sprayed on the tablecloths and napkins, diffused in the air. The guests each got a bottle to take home, too. Everyone got to take part in something that meant a lot to Nicole, her mother, and me. What's more, they would remember the wedding every time they reexperienced that smell.

I took the fragrance theme even one step further and put a little personal stamp of my own on the affair. At the end of the reception, I had a helicopter drop thousands of rose petals on the crowd. No one at that wedding will ever forget that the bride's father does *something* having to do with *real* plant and flower essences, now will they?

AROMATIC MOMENTS REVISITED

Flowers and weddings—and celebrations of all kinds—have a long-lasting history together. In Bali, for example, before a couple is married, they each

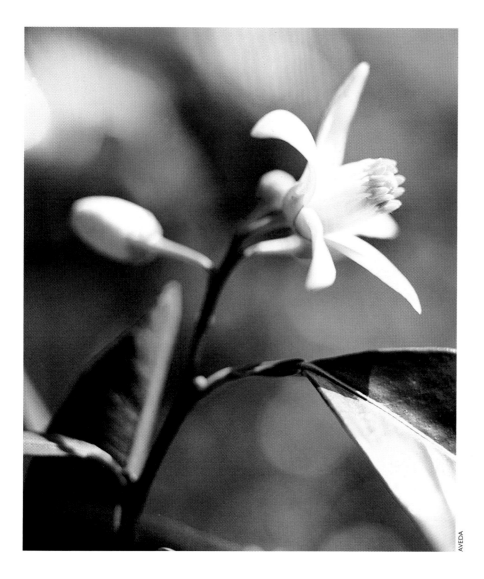

AVEDA

Don't forget beautiful scents, like neroli, to help heighten joyful days.

take part in an ancient ritual called a *lulur* bath, a ceremonial dousing in warm, fragrant water filled with frangipani flowers. In India, at Ayurvedic wedding ceremonies, fresh rose water is sprayed all over everything and used in the wedding ceremony.

Special aromatics like these are a wonderful way to make all important occasions even more memorable. Sense memory allows us to recapture the feelings of certain moments every time we present our olfactory systems with that same chemical data. Give your child a combination of essential oils to wear or breathe at a first Holy Communion or bar or bat mitzvah, and, for years to come, he or she will remember that day every time that scent is present nearby. Choose a plant-based fragrance that you and your partner both love, include it in a special occasion, like your wedding, and that fragrance will always bring you both back to the mood of that special day.

A LINGERING, SWEET SMELL

One of the great mysteries of relationships is how to keep renewing them and recapturing those first feelings of early love. Aromatics can play a great role in this quest for partnership rejuvenation. They can bring us back to a time, place, and a mood. If you get married, I recommend taking the scent from your wedding day on the honeymoon to keep the feeling of that big day along for the ride. That scent can be an essence that's the same as the flowers from your wedding, or a combination of essential oils you both choose beforehand to spray and dab around the room. Bring that fragrance out again and again, for anniversaries and other special occasions. It will always give you good sense memory responses. (It may also come in handy on the rare occasions you have a fight and need to kiss and make up!)

I believe that when couples are about to get married or move in together, almost as important as registering for wedding gifts and shopping for furniture is taking a sensory journey together to discover which aromas they both enjoy, and which ones arouse certain moods and feelings. The sensory journey itself can be a special occasion, a day of togetherness and celebration of the relationship, which you repeat every year or so to broaden your fragrance horizons. Once you find a few favorites, use them regularly; but also bring them into your special celebrations to help you mark the occasions in your minds, and your olfactory systems. You'll be creating a library in your brain that you can easily access with just a little whiff of your signature essential oil combinations.

PRIVATE PRACTICE

Regardless of the occasion, we can better prepare ourselves, emotionally and physically, by giving ourselves some special treatments now and then. These occasions are also a good excuse to touch down with some of the coaches and practitioners in various sectors of our lives.

▶ Treat yourself to a professional massage, facial, or other spa treatment once a month, or as often as you can afford it. Do these as a treat before special, rare occasions like a wedding. These rituals can be helpful in cleansing us before we make life changes, like entering into marriage. Cleansing rituals are also good to engage in after a death has occurred. That's a way of attaching a fresh beginning to an ending.

▶ See your doctors at least once a year, and visit your dentist for a cleaning and checkup.

▶ Take a class in healthy cooking.

▶ If you work out alone at home, go to an exercise or yoga class occasionally to come into contact with others and with teachers who can remind us of the right ways to do things.

▶ Attend a meditational *Satsang*, or chanting ceremony, at a local yoga studio to align your meditation with others. Or, perhaps spend a weekend at an ashram or other place of retreat where you can recharge your batteries.

▶ Disappear into the Himalayas, or to a tepee, for ten days of silence, including five days of near-fasting. That is one of my favorite ways of cleansing myself in all sectors of my being and of taking stock each year.

TIME-HONORED TRADITIONS

Our religions and cultures provide many rituals concerning holidays and special occasions. There are times to fast, times to cleanse, times to omit certain foods from our diets. These customs usually have their roots in some sound wisdom regarding health and spirituality. For example, the Christian holiday of Lent, during which many people avoid eating meat, takes place in the spring, a perfect time for dietary cleansing after a hearty winter. Orthodox Jewish women go to a *mikvah,* or ceremonial bathhouse, at the end of their menstrual periods to cleanse themselves physically and spiritually. The Jewish faith also has five annual days of fasting, providing cleansing opportunities interspersed throughout the calendar year.

Many traditions also have rituals associated with renewal following death. In Bali, a funeral is a celebration, filled with offerings to the gods to help the deceased move on to the next life happily and peacefully. I like to use essential oils I love during times of grieving to help uplift my spirits.

I recommend exploring your own heritage as well as others for established customs that will lend meaning to your special days. And I suggest that you use your imagination and the things you have learned about your own sense of pleasure through your personal inventory to create new rituals of your own to commemorate times of celebration and change in your life.

Glossary of Essential Oils

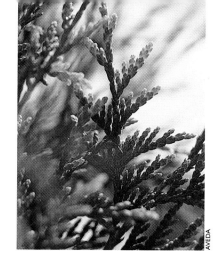

AMYRIS OIL

Source: Amyris
Description: Pale yellow straw color,
  clear oily liquid
Part Used: Wood
Preparation Method: Steam distillation
Olfactory Description: Woody; balsamic,
  slightly woody, with sweetish floral
  undernote
Blends Well With: Cedarwood,
  citronella, lavandin, oakmoss
Perfumery Note: Middle-base
Aromatherapy Classification: Energizing
Ayurvedic Classification:
  Kapha or earth/water
Flash Point: 230° F.
Safety: Nonflammable; not known as a
  skin irritant; possibly orally toxic
Storage: Room temperature
Aromatherapy Applications:
  Grounding, energizing, tonifying,
  balancing
Skin Care Application: Blemished skin,
  dry skin, waterlogged skin
AVEDA Products: Purescriptions—Dry
  Remedy, Elixir Remedy—and other
  products

ANISE OIL

Source: Anise seed
Description: Colorless to pale yellow,
  clear thin liquid
Part Used: Seeds
Preparation Method: Steam distillation
Olfactory Description: Anise note;
  extremely sweet, smooth, and clean
  warm note; somewhat with
  herbaceous undernote
Blends Well With: Amyris, bay, caraway,
  cardamom, cedarwood, coriander,
  dill, fennel, galbanum, mandarin,
  petitgrain, rosewood
Perfumery Note: Top-middle
Aromatherapy Classification: Energizing
Ayurvedic Classification:
  Kapha or earth/water
Flash Point: 182° F.
Safety: Slight dermal toxicity; use
  ½ recommended dilution or less
Storage: Refrigerate
Aromatherapy Applications: Energizing,
  tonifying
Skin Care Application: Not used
AVEDA Products: Indigenous Pure-
  fume—Hana Spirit; Key Element 15
  water nature (Aroma); Shampure;
  and other products

BASIL OIL, ORGANIC

Source: Basil
Description: Light yellow iridescent,
  clear aromatic oily liquid
Part Used: Leaves
Preparation Method: Steam distillation
Olfactory Description: Anise note; sweet
  floral, spicy, with aniselike undertones
Blends Well With: Bergamot, black
  pepper, clary sage, geranium, hyssop,
  lavender, marjoram, neroli,
  sandalwood, verbena
Perfumery Note: Top-middle
Aromatherapy Classification: Calming
Ayurvedic Classification:
  Kapha or earth/water
Flash Point: 107° F.
Safety: Use ½ recommended dilution or
  less; low potential for skin irritation;
  slight to moderate toxicity orally
Storage: Refrigerate
Aromatherapy Application:
  Soothing, energizing, tonifying,
  breath-freshening
Skin Care Application: Oily skin,
  waterlogged skin. Note: Toxic—
  use ½ recommended dilution
AVEDA Products: Key Element 3 fire
  nature (Aroma) and other products

BAY OIL

Source: Bay leaf

Description: Clear yellow to brownish yellow, mobile liquid

Part Used: Leaves

Preparation Method: Steam distillation

Olfactory Description: Spice note; warm, somewhat fennel-like sweet, spicy, with reminiscence of metallic impression

Blends Well With: Cedarwood, coriander, eucalyptus, ginger, juniper, lavender, lemon, marjoram, orange, rose, rosemary, thyme, ylang-ylang

Perfumery Note: Top-middle

Aromatherapy Classification: Energizing

Ayurvedic Classification: Vata or air

Flash Point: 115° F.

Safety: Use ½ recommended dilution or less; can cause skin irritation

Storage: Refrigerate

Aromatherapy Applications: Stimulating, energizing

Skin Care Application: Not used

AVEDA Products: Indigenous Pure-fume—Mizan Absolute, Mizan Spirit—and other products

BERGAMOT OIL

Source: Bergamot

Description: Clear yellow to green, oily liquid

Part Used: Fruit peels

Preparation Method: Expression

Olfactory Description: Fresh, citrus-sweet, fruity

Blends Well With: Chamomile, coriander, cypress, geranium, juniper, lavender, lemon, neroli, ylang-ylang

Perfumery Note: Citrus

Aromatherapy Classification: Calming

Ayurvedic Classification: Vata or air

Flash Point: 144° F.

Safety: Nontoxic, nonirritant, nonphototoxic, nonsensitizing

Storage: Refrigerate

Aromatherapy Applications: Calming, tonic, deodorizing, balancing

Skin Care Application: Blemished skin, Normal/combination skin, oily skin

AVEDA Products: All Chakra III products; Indigenous Pure-fume—Isesi Absolute, Isesi Spirit; Love; Singular Notes—Bergamot; and other products

BLACK PEPPER OIL

Source: Pepper

Description: Very pale yellow to pale yellow, clear mobile aromatic oily liquid

Part Used: Fruits

Preparation Method: Steam distillation

Olfactory Description: Spice note; sharp, spicy, slightly herbaceous undertones

Blends Well With: Lavender, marjoram, olibanum, rosemary, sandalwood

Perfumery Note: Top-middle

Aromatherapy Classification: Energizing

Ayurvedic Classification: Kapha or earth/water

Flash Point: 107° F.

Safety: Undiluted oil may be irritating to skin and eyes; orally toxic

Storage: Refrigerate

Aromatherapy Applications: Tonifying

Skin Care Application: Not used

AVEDA Products: Annatto color conditioners—Bixa, Black Malva, Blue Malva, Camomile, Clove, Madder Root—and other products

CAJEPUT OIL

Source: Cajeput

Description: Colorless to pale green yellow, clear oily liquid

Parts Used: Leaves and stems

Preparation Method: Steam distillation

Olfactory Description: Camphoraceous; medicinal, camphoraceous, and very penetrating; reminiscent of eucalyptus

Blends Well With: Angelica, bergamot, birch, cardamom, clove, geranium, imortelle, lavender, myrtle, niaouli, nutmeg, rose, rosewood, thyme

Perfumery Note: Top-middle

Aromatherapy Classification: Energizing

Ayurvedic Classification: Vata or air

Flash Point: 120° F.

Safety: Highly toxic orally

Storage: Refrigerate

Aromatherapy Applications: Soothing, stimulating, energizing

Skin Care Applications: Blemished skin, waterlogged skin

AVEDA Products: Active Composition and other products

CARAWAY SEED OIL

Source: Caraway

Description: Clear, colorless to pale yellow, limpid oily liquid

Part Used: Seeds

Preparation Method: Steam distillation

Olfactory Description: Minty; clean, fresh, spicy, with earthy undernote

Blends Well With: Eucalyptus, fir needle absolute, galbanum, pine, rosemary

Perfumery Note: Top-middle

Aromatherapy Classification: Energizing

Ayurvedic Classification: Kapha or earth/water

Flash Point: 120° F.

Safety: Slight dermal toxicity

Storage: Refrigerate

Aromatherapy Application: Stimulating

Skin Care Application: Not used

AVEDA Products: All Chakra VI products; all Chakra VII products; Indigenous Pure-fume—Eros Absolute, Eros Spirit; and other products

CARDAMOM OIL

Source: Cardamom

Description: Colorless to pale yellow, clear aromatic oily liquid

Part Used: Seeds

Preparation Method: Steam distillation

Olfactory Description: Spice note; warm, earthy, spicy, with hint of fishy undernote

Blends Well With: Coriander,

frankincense, galbanum, geranium, juniper, lemon, myrtle, pine, verbena
Perfumery Note: Middle-base
Aromatherapy Classification: Energizing
Ayurvedic Classification:
    Kapha or earth/water
Flash Point: 129° F.
Safety: Undiluted oil may cause skin irritation
Storage: Refrigerate
Aromatherapy Applications: Stimulating, tonifying, skin cleanser
Skin Care Application: Not used
AVEDA Products: All Chakra I products, all Chakra V products, and other products

CARROT SEED OIL

Source: Carrot seed
Description: Light yellow to amber, clear aromatic oily liquid
Part Used: Seeds
Preparation Method: Steam distillation
Olfactory Description: Spice note; penetrating clean, dry, fresh note, with warm earthy undernote
Blends Well With: Bergamot, juniper, lavender, lemon, lime, melissa, neroli, orange, petitgrain, rosemary, verbena
Perfumery Note: Top-middle
Aromatherapy Classification: Energizing
Ayurvedic Classification:
    Kapha or earth/water
Flash Point: 117° F.
Safety: Undiluted oil may be irritating to skin and eyes
Storage: Refrigerate
Aromatherapy Applications: Stimulating, tonifying
Skin Care Applications: All types, dry skin, inflamed skin, mature skin, normal/combination skin. Note: Anticoagulant. Note: Toxic—use ½ recommended dilution
AVEDA Products: All Chakra IV products; Indigenous Pure-fume— Gaia Absolute, Gaia Spirit, Mizan Absolute, Mizan Spirit; and other products

CEDARWOOD OIL

Source: Cedarwood, Moroccan
Description: Light yellow to pale brown, clear aromatic oily liquid
Part Used: Wood
Preparation Method: Steam distillation
Olfactory Description: Woody; oily woody, typical of cedarwood balsamic odor, reminiscent of the pencil note
Blends Well With: Patchouli, sandalwood, vetiver
Perfumery Note: Top-middle
Aromatherapy Classification: Energizing
Ayurvedic Classification:
    Kapha or earth/water
Flash Point: 200° F.
Safety: Nontoxic, very mild skin irritant, nonsensitizing, nonphototoxic
Storage: Store in cool, dry area in closed containers; do not expose to high temperatures.
Aromatherapy Applications: Skin conditioner, deodorant, insect repellent, soothing agent
Skin Care Application: Blemished skin
AVEDA Products: All Chakra I products, Rainforest Aroma Mist, Rainforest Candle, and other products

CELERY SEED OIL

Source: Celery seed
Description: Yellow to greenish brown color, clear thin liquid
Part Used: Seeds
Preparation Method: Steam distillation
Olfactory Description: Spice note; spicy warm, with hint of penetrating, dry, granular note
Blends Well With: Angelica, basil, cajeput, chamomile, grapefruit, guaiacwood, lemon, orange, palmarosa, rosemary, verbena
Perfumery Note: Top-middle
Aromatherapy Classification: Energizing
Ayurvedic Classification: Vata or air

Flash Point: 120° F.
Safety: Undiluted oil may be irritating to skin and eyes. Note: Toxic—use ½ recommended dilution
Storage: Refrigerate
Aromatherapy Applications: Stimulating, tonifying
Skin Care Applications: Not used
AVEDA Products: All Chakra II products; Indigenous Pure-fume— Psyche Absolute, Psyche Spirit; Rainforest Candle; and other products

CHAMOMILE OIL

Source: Chamomile, blue
Description: Dark blue, clear liquid
Part Used: Flowers
Preparation Method: Steam distillation
Olfactory Description: Fruity; tenaciously sweet, with floral herbaceous and bitter undernote
Blends Well With: Bergamot, clary sage, jasmine, labdanum, neroli, oakmoss, rose
Perfumery Note: Middle-base
Aromatherapy Classification: Calming
Ayurvedic Classification:
    Kapha or earth/water
Flash Point: 123° F.
Safety: Undiluted oil may be irritating to skin and eyes
Storage: Refrigerate
Aromatherapy Applications: Soothing, tonifying
Skin Care Applications: Dry skin, inflamed skin, normal/combination skin, sensitive skin. Note: Cicatrizing or cytophylactic
AVEDA Products: Skin Firming/Toning Agent and other products

CHAMOMILE OIL, SAUVAGE

Source: Chamomile, Moroccan
Description: Clear yellow to amber, oily aromatic liquid
Part Used: Flowering tops

CHAMOMILE OIL, SAUVAGE *(continued)*

Preparation Method: Steam distillation

Olfactory Description: Aromatic; mild, sweet, fresh hint of citrus, with earthy warmth

Blends Well With: Artemesia, cedarwood, cypress, labdanum, lavindin, lavender, oakmoss, olibanum, vetiver

Perfumery Note: Middle-base

Aromatherapy Classification: Calming

Ayurvedic Classification: Kapha or earth/water

Flash Point: 125° F.

Safety: OK

Storage: Refrigerate

Aromatherapy Applications: Balancing, soothing, calming, tonifying

Skin Care Applications: Dry skin, inflamed skin, normal/combination skin, sensitive skin

AVEDA Products: Exfoliant; Hydrating Lotion; Purifying Creme Cleanser; Purifying Gel Cleanser; Purifying Waters—Camomile; Singular Notes—Camomile; and other products

CHAMOMILE OIL

Source: Chamomile, Roman

Description: Pale yellow, clear oily liquid

Part Used: Flowers

Preparation Method: Steam distillation

Olfactory Description: Fruity; bittersweet, warm, herbaceous, with fruity, tea leaflike undertones, also a hint of powdery note

Blends Well With: Eucalyptus, fir needle absolute, galbanum, pine, rosemary

Perfumery Note: Middle-base

Aromatherapy Classification: Calming

Ayurvedic Classification: Kapha or earth/water

Flash Point: 125° F.

Safety: Nontoxic, very mild irritant, nonphototoxic, nonsensitizing

Storage: Refrigerate

Aromatherapy Applications: Calming, tonifying

Skin Care Applications: Dry skin, inflamed skin, normal/combination, skin, sensitive skin

AVEDA Products: All Chakra VI products; all Chakra VII products; Indigenous Pure-fume—Isesi Absolute, Isesi Spirit; and other products

CISTUS OIL

Source: Labdanum

Description: Light orange, clear mobile liquid

Part Used: Resin

Preparation Method: Steam distillation

Olfactory Description: Balsamic; sweet, herbaceous-green, balsamic with amberlike undernote

Blends Well With: Bergamot, clary sage, cypress, juniper, lavender, oakmoss, olibanum, patchouli, pine, sandalwood, vetiver

Perfumery Note: Middle-base

Aromatherapy Classification: Calming

Ayurvedic Classification: Vata or air

Flash Point: 149° F.

Safety: Nontoxic, nonirritant, nonphototoxic, nonsensitizing

Storage: Refrigerate

Aromatherapy Applications: Stimulating, tonifying, soothing

Skin Care Applications: Inflamed skin, mature skin, sensitive skin. Note: Skin conditioning. Note: Toxic—use ½ recommended dilution

AVEDA Products: All Chakra II products; all Chakra VI products; Key Element—1 earth nature (Aroma), 6 water air nature; and other products

CITRONELLA OIL

Source: Citronella

Description: Light yellow to amber, clear aromatic oily liquid

Parts Used: Aerial parts

Preparation Method: Steam distillation

Olfactory Description: Citrus; very fresh citrus note, with hint of roselike topnote

Blends Well With: Bergamot, lemon, lemongrass, melissa, orange

Perfumery Note: Top-middle

Aromatherapy Classification: Energizing

Ayurvedic Classification: Vata or air

Flash Point: 175° F.

Safety: Undiluted oil may be irritating to skin, eyes, and mucous membranes; low toxicity potential

Storage: Room temperature

Aromatherapy Application: Soothing

Skin Care Application: Skin conditioning

AVEDA Products: Firmata; Indigenous Pure-fume—Hana Absolute, Hana Spirit; Purifying Mist—Attracts Humans, Not Insects; and other products

CLARY SAGE OIL

Source: Sage, Clary

Description: Pale yellow to yellow, clear liquid

Part Used: Flowering tops

Preparation Method: Steam distillation

Olfactory Description: Herbaceous; smooth herbaceous with tenacious sweetness, reminiscent of balsamic note

Blends Well With: Cedarwood, citrus, labdanum, lavindin, lavender, musks

Perfumery Note: Top-middle

Aromatherapy Classification: Calming

Ayurvedic Classification: Kapha or earth/water

Flash Point: 125° F.

Safety: Use ⅓ recommended dilution or less

Storage: Refrigerate

Aromatherapy Applications: Balancing, calming, tonifying

Skin Care Applications: Dry skin, inflamed skin, mature skin, normal/combination skin

AVEDA Products: Calming Hand & Body Shower/Bath Cleanser; Cherry/Almond Bark Rejuvenating

Conditioner; Body Compounds—Chi, Relax; Cleansers—Chi, Relax, Total Body; Lavandou Candle; Purifying Mist—Insightful; Shampoos—Black Malva, Blue Malva, Camomile, Clove, Madder Root; and other products

CLOVE BUD OIL

Source: Clove
Description: Clear colorless to pale yellow liquid
Part Used: Flowers
Preparation Method: Steam distillation
Olfactory Description: Spice note; warm sweet-spicy aroma, truly reminiscent of the dried buds
Blends Well With: Basil, benzoin, black pepper, cinnamon, citronella, grapefruit, lemon, nutmeg, orange, peppermint, rosemary, rose
Perfumery Note: Top-middle-base
Aromatherapy Classification: Energizing
Ayurvedic Classification: Pitta or fire
Flash Point: >200° F.
Safety: Use ½ recommended dilution or less; can cause skin irritation
Storage: Room temperature
Aromatherapy Applications: Stimulating, energizing
Skin Care Applications: Not used
Note: Potential toxicity—use ½ recommended dilution
AVEDA Products: Key Element 15 water nature (Aroma); Singular Notes—Cinnamon; and other products

CORIANDER OIL

Source: Coriander
Description: Clear to pale yellow liquid
Part Used: Seeds
Preparation Method: Steam distillation
Olfactory Description: Spice note; pleasant, sweet, somewhat woody/spicy
Blends Well With: Bergamot, black

pepper, cinnamon, citronella, cypress, galbanum, ginger, jasmine, lemon, melissa, neroli, orange
Perfumery Note: Top-middle
Aromatherapy Classification: Energizing
Ayurvedic Classifications: Kapha or earth/water, pitta or fire, vata or air
Flash Point: 167° F.
Safety: Undiluted oil may be irritating to skin and eyes
Storage: Refrigerate
Aromatherapy Applications: Warming, tonic, stimulating, antimicrobial (preserving)
Skin Care Application: Not used
AVEDA Products: Adaptive Bath Essence Base; Attar Absolute; Calming Composition; all Chakra I products; all Chakra VII products; Curessence; Indigenous Pure-fume—Psyche Absolute, Psyche Spirit; Key Element 6 water air nature; Potpourri—Rose; Rainforest Aroma Diffuser Oil; Styling Curessence; and other products

CYPRESS OIL

Source: Cypress
Description: Light yellow color, clear oily liquid
Parts Used: Leaves and stems
Preparation Method: Steam distillation
Olfactory Description: Coniferous; fresh pinelike woody-balsamic, with spicy, cirtus undernote
Blends Well With: Benzoin, bergamot, clary sage, juniper, lavender, lemon, orange, pine, rosemary, sandalwood
Perfumery Note: Top-middle
Aromatherapy Classification: Energizing
Ayurvedic Classifications: Pitta or fire, vata or air
Flash Point: 95° F.
Safety: Nontoxic, very mild irritant, nonphototoxic, nonsensitizing
Storage: Refrigerate
Aromatherapy Applications: Stimulating, cleansing, antimicrobial (preserving), astringent

Skin Care Applications: Blemished skin, oily skin, waterlogged skin
AVEDA Products: Pure-fume Brilliant—Anti-Humectant Pomade, Emollient For Hair, Forming Gel, Humectant Pomade—and other products

ELEMI OIL

Source: Elemi
Description: Pale yellow-green, clear yellowish liquid
Part Used: Resin
Preparation Method: Steam distillation
Olfactory Description: Citrus; peppery-citrus characteristic
Blends Well With: Citrus oils, cinnamon bark, cistus, labdanum, lavender, olibanum, rosemary, sage
Perfumery Note: Top-middle
Aromatherapy Classifications: Calming
Ayurvedic Classifications: Vata or air
Flash Point: 111° F.
Safety: Slightly toxic orally; undiluted oil may be irritating to skin and eyes
Storage: Room temperature
Aromatherapy Applications: Stimulating, soothing, skin conditioning, antimicrobial (preserving)
Skin Care Application: Skin conditioning
AVEDA Products: Indigenous Pure-fume—Isesi Absolute, Isesi Spirit; Potpourri—Spice; and other products

EUCALYPTUS OIL

Source: Eucalyptus (Blue Gum)
Description: Pale yellow, clear liquid
Parts Used: Leaves and stems
Preparation Method: Steam distillation
Olfactory Description: Camphoraceous; fresh light camphoraceous, with touch of medicinal undertone
Blends Well With: Benzoin, coriander, juniper, lavender, lemon, lemongrass, melissa, pine, thyme
Perfumery Note: Top-middle

EUCALYPTUS OIL *(continued)*
Aromatherapy Classification: Energizing
Ayurvedic Classification:
    Kapha or earth/water
Flash Point: 120° F.
Safety: Nonirritating, nonsensitizing,
    nonphototoxic; orally toxic; keep out
    of reach of children
Storage: Room temperature
Aromatherapy Applications:
    Tonifying, stimulating, antimicrobial
    (preserving)
Skin Care Application: Blemished skin
AVEDA Products: Active Composition;
    Color Conditioners—Annatto, Bixa,
    Black Malva, Blue Malva, Camomile,
    Clove, Madder Root; Key Element—
    2 water nature (Aroma), 12 earth
    nature (Aroma); Lavandou Candle;
    Potpourri—Lavender; Purifying
    Mist—Nurturing; Singular Notes—
    Eucalyptus; and other products

FENNEL OIL, SWEET

Source: Fennel
Description: Colorless to slightly yellow,
    clear mobile oily iridescent liquid
Part Used: Fruits
Preparation Method: Steam distillation
Olfactory Description: Anise note;
    sweet, floral, with herbaceous spicy
    undernote, reminiscent of anise
Blends Well With: Basil, geranium,
    lavender, lemon, rose, rosemary,
    sandalwood
Perfumery Note: Top-middle
Aromatherapy Classification: Energizing
Ayurvedic Classification:
    Kapha or earth/water
Flash Point: 180° F.
Safety: Slight dermal toxicity; use
    ½ recommended dilution or less
Storage: Refrigerate
Aromatherapy Applications: Energizing,
    tonifying
Skin Care Applications: Waterlogged
    skin. Note: Anticoagulant. Note:
    Toxic—use ½ recommended dilution
AVEDA Products: All Chakra I

products, Miraculous Beauty
Replenisher, and other products

GALBANUM OIL

Source: Galbanum
Description: Light yellow, clear liquid
Part Used: Resin
Preparation Method: Steam distillation
Olfactory Description: Green; intensely
    leafy-green aroma with woody
    undernote
Blends Well With: Citronella, elemi,
    frankincense, geranium, ginger,
    jasmine, palmarosa, pine, rose,
    tagetes verbena, ylang-ylang
Perfumery Note: Top-middle
Aromatherapy Classification: Energizing
Ayurvedic Classification: Vata or air
Flash Point: 104° F.
Safety: Undiluted oil may cause
    irritation to skin and eyes
Storage: Refrigerate
Aromatherapy Applications: Tonifying,
    stimulating
Skin Care Applications: Blemished skin.
    Note: Skin conditioning. Note:
    Anticoagulant
AVEDA Products: Key Element 8 air
    water fire nature, all Pure-fume
    Brilliant products, and other products

GERANIUM OIL BOURBON

Source: Geranium
Description: Clear, colorless, sometimes
    faint green-olive to a brownish green,
    limpid liquid
Parts Used: Leaves and stems
Preparation Method: Steam distillation
Olfactory Description: Floral; minty-
    fruity topnote, with strong leaflike
    rosy undertones
Blends Well With: Angelica, basil, bay,
    bergamot, carrot seed, cedarwood,
    citronella, clary sage, grapefruit,
    jasmine, lavender, lime, neroli,
    orange, petitgrain, rose, rosemary,
    sandalwood
Perfumery Note: Top-middle-base

Aromatherapy Classification: Calming
Ayurvedic Classification: Pitta or fire
Flash Point: 179° F.
Safety: Slight dermal toxicity
Storage: Refrigerate
Aromatherapy Applications: Balancing,
    tonifying, soothing
Skin Care Applications: All types,
    blemished skin, dry skin, inflamed
    skin, normal/combination, oily skin,
    waterlogged skin. Note: Toxic—use
    ½ recommended dilution
AVEDA Products: All All-Sensitive
    products; Exfoliant; Hydrating Lotion;
    Indigenous Pure-fume—Gaia Absolute;
    Key Element 2 water nature (Aroma);
    all Pure-fume Brilliant products;
    Purescriptions—Dry Remedy, Elixir
    Remedy, Oily Remedy; Purifying
    Creme Cleanser; Purifying Gel
    Cleanser; and other products

GINGER OIL

Source: Ginger
Description: Very pale yellow to light
    amber, mobile liquid
Part Used: Roots
Preparation Method: Steam distillation
Olfactory Description: Spicy note; spicy,
    sharp, warm, and pleasant; very alive,
    with hint of lemon and pepper
Blends Well With: Bay, cajuput,
    caraway, cardamom, cinnamon,
    clove, coriander, elemi, eucalyptus,
    frankincense, geranium, lemon,
    lime, myrtle, orange, rosemary,
    spearmint, verbena
Perfumery Note: Top-middle
Aromatherapy Classification: Energizing
Ayurvedic Classification: Vata or air
Flash Point: 130° F.
Safety: Undiluted oil may be irritating to
    skin and eyes
Storage: Refrigerate
Aromatherapy Applications: Energizing,
    tonifying, warming
Skin Care Application: Not used
AVEDA Products: Indigenous
    Pure-fume—Amazonia Absolute,

Amazonia Spirit; Key Element 29 full spectrum (Aroma); Shave Emollient; and other products

GRAPEFRUIT OIL

Source: Grapefruit

Description: Colorless to slightly orange, clear liquid

Part Used: Fruit peels

Preparation Method: Expression

Olfactory Description: Citrus; sweet, sharp citrus, bitter floral and refreshing

Blends Well With: Citrus oils, especially with bergamot and orange

Perfumery Note: Top

Aromatherapy Classification: Energizing

Ayurvedic Classification: Vata or air

Flash Point: 111° F.

Safety: Undiluted oil may be irritating to skin and eyes

Storage: Refrigerate

Aromatherapy Applications: Energizing, air refreshening

Skin Care Applications: Waterlogged skin. Note: Toxic—use ½ recommended dilution

AVEDA Products: Bio-Molecular Perfecting Fluid; Cherry/Almond Bark Rejuvenating Conditioner; Shampoos—Black Malva, Blue Malva, Camomile, Clove, Madder Root, Pro; Purifying Mist—Arise, Insightful; Shave Emollient; and other products

JASMIN ABSOLUTE

Source: Jasmine, Arabian

Description: Medium to dark amber, clear liquid

Part Used: Flowers

Preparation Method: Solvent extraction

Olfactory Description: Floral; intensely floral, honeylike sweet, warm, with herbaceous-fruity undertones

Blends Well With: virtually all of the floral absolutes, i.e., cassie, genet, mimosa, rose, ylang-ylang

Perfumery Note: Top-middle-base

Aromatherapy Classification: Energizing

Ayurvedic Classifications: Kapha or earth/water, Pitta or fire, Vata or air

Flash Point: 138° F.

Safety: Nontoxic, nonirritant, nonphototoxic, nonsensitizing

Storage: Cool area, away from heat and flames, in containers that are closed and plainly labeled

Aromatherapy Applications: Antiseptic, aphrodisiac, soothing agent

Skin Care Application: All types

AVEDA Products: All Chakra II products; all Chakra V products; all Chakra VI products; all Chakra VII products; Color Concentrate—Dark Brown/Brun fonce 2, Neutral Blonde/Blond neute 11; Elixir; Euphoric—Aroma Mist, Diffuser Oil; Hydrating Lotion; Key Element—3 fire nature (Aroma), 4 air nature, 5 infinity nature, 9 water air fire nature; Madagascar Candle; Purifying Creme Cleanser; Purifying Gel Cleanser; Purifying Mist—Euphoric; Purifying Waters—Jasmine; and Valencia Candle

JUNIPER BERRY OIL

Source: Juniper berry

Description: Light yellow to pale yellow color, clear oily liquid

Part Used: Fruits

Preparation Method: Steam distillation

Olfactory Description: Coniferous; sweet woody, with pine needlelike undernote, with reminiscence of gin

Blends Well With: Benzoin resinoid, clary sage, cypress, elemi, fir needle, lavindin, lovage, oakmoss, opoponax

Perfumery Note: Top-middle

Aromatherapy Classification: Energizing

Ayurvedic Classifications: Pitta or fire, vata or air

Flash Point: 99° F.

Safety: Flammable; slightly irritating to skin; should always be used diluted

Storage: Refrigerate

Aromatherapy Applications: Energizing, antimicrobial (preserving), astringent

Skin Care Applications: Blemished skin, oily skin, waterlogged skin. Note: Toxic—use ½ recommended dilution

AVEDA Products: Indigenous Pure-fume—Amazonia Absolute, Amazonia Spirit; Key Element 8 air water fire nature; and other products

LAVANDIN ABRIALIS OIL

Source: Lavandin

Description: Pale yellow to yellow-green color, clear mobile liquid

Part Used: Leaves

Preparation Method: Steam distillation

Olfactory Description: Herbaceous; fresh, woody, spicy, camphoraceous lavender

Blends Well With: Bay leaf, cinnamon leaf, clove, citronella, cypress, geranium, origanum, patchouli, pine needle

Perfumery Note: Top-middle

Aromatherapy Classification: Energizing

Ayurvedic Classification: Vata or air

Flash Point: 132° F.

Safety: Undiluted oil may be irritating to skin and eyes

Storage: Refrigerate

Aromatherapy Applications: Stimulating, energizing, antimicrobial (preserving), tonifying

Skin Care Application: Skin conditioning. Note: Potential toxicity—use ½ recommended dilution

AVEDA Products: Indigenous Pure-fume—Amazonia Absolute, Amazonia Spirit; Shave Emollient; and other products

LAVENDER FLEURS OIL

Source: Lavender

Description: Clear colorless to light yellow, oily liquid

Part Used: Flowering tops

Preparation Method: Steam distillation

LAVENDER FLEURS OIL (*continued*)

Olfactory Description: Herbaceous; very refreshing, smooth, sweet, floral, with herbaceous undertone

Blends Well With: Bergamot, clary sage, clove, eucalyptus, jasmine, oakmoss, patchouli, pine, rose, rosemary

Perfumery Note: Top-middle

Aromatherapy Classification: Calming

Ayurvedic Classifications: Vata or air

Flash Point: 165° F.

Safety: Nonirritating, nonsensitizing, nonphototoxic

Storage: Refrigerate

Aromatherapy Applications: Calming, antimicrobial; an all-purpose oil; with right dosage, can be used for almost any condition

Skin Care Applications: All types, dry skin, inflamed skin, normal/combination skin, oily skin, sensitive skin, waterlogged skin

AVEDA Products: Active Composition; Beautifying Formula; Calming Hand & Body Shower/Bath Cleanser; all Chakra III products; Color Conditioners—Annato, Bixa, Black Malva, Blue Malva, Camomile, Clove, Madder Root; Key Element 25 infinity nature (Aroma); Lavandou Aroma Diffuser Oil; Lavandou Aroma Mist; Miraculous Beauty Replenisher; Potpourri—Lavender; Purescriptions Elixir Remedy; Purescriptions Oily Remedy; Purifying Mist—Arise, Nurturing; Purifying Waters—Lavender; Self-Timing Perm; Singular Notes—Lavender Fleurs; and other products

SPIKE LAVENDER OIL

Source: Lavender, spike

Description: Clear pale yellow to yellow, oily mobile liquid

Part Used: Flowering tops

Preparation Method: Steam distillation

Olfactory Description: Herbaceous; sharp, camphoraceous, lavenderlike.

Blends Well With: Bois de rose,

eucalyptus, lavandin, lavender, neroli, petitgrain, rosemary

Perfumery Note: Top-middle

Aromatherapy Classification: Energizing

Ayurvedic Classification: Vata or air

Flash Point: 131° F.

Safety: Slightly toxic orally, dermally

Storage: Room temperature

Aromatherapy Applications: Stimulating, energizing, antimicrobial (preserving), tonifying

Skin Care Applications: Inflamed skin, mature skin, normal/combination skin, oily skin. Note: Skin conditioning

AVEDA Products: Lavandou Candle; Potpourri—Lavender; Purifying Mist—Attracts Humans, Not Insects; and other products

LEMON OIL

Source: Lemon

Description: Pale yellow to greenish yellow, clear thin liquid

Part Used: Fruit peels

Preparation Method: Expression

Olfactory Description: Citrus; fresh, light, outdoorsy aroma, characteristic of lemon

Blends Well With: Bergamot, citronella, clary sage, galbanum, neroli, orange flower, violet leaf

Perfumery Note: Top

Aromatherapy Classification: Energizing

Ayurvedic Classification: Vata or air

Flash Point: 115° F.

Safety: Undiluted oil may be irritating to skin and eyes; prolonged or repeated contact may cause skin irritation; may produce phototoxic effects, should always be substantially diluted

Storage: Refrigerate

Aromatherapy Applications: Energizing, uplifting

Skin Care Applications: Blemished skin, normal/combination skin, oily skin. Note: Anticoagulant

AVEDA Products: After Shave Balm; Bio-Molecular Perfecting Fluid;

Key Element—1 earth nature (Aroma), 7 air water nature, 29 full spectrum (Aroma); Sunsource; Valencia Aroma Mist; Vital Elements Fabric Cleanser; and other products

LEMONGRASS OIL

Source: Lemongrass

Description: Clear colorless to pale yellow, mobile liquid

Parts Used: Aerial parts

Preparation Method: Steam distillation

Olfactory Description: Citrus; strong lemon note, with sweet herbaceous undertone

Blends Well With: Geranium, jasmine, lavender

Perfumery Note: Top-middle

Aromatherapy Classification: Calming

Ayurvedic Classification: Pitta or fire

Flash Point: 167° F.

Safety: Can cause skin irritation; mildly toxic

Storage: Refrigerate

Aromatherapy Applications: Calming, antimicrobial (preserving)

Skin Care Applications: Blemished skin, mature skin, oily skin. Note: Toxic— use ½ recommended dilution

AVEDA Products: Color Conditioners— Annatto, Bixa, Black Malva, Blue Malva, Camomile, Clove, Madder Root—and other products

LIME OIL

Source: Lime

Description: Colorless to greenish yellow, clear mobile aromatic liquid

Part Used: Fruit peels

Preparation Method: Steam distillation

Olfactory Description: Citrus; fresh, sharp, sweet citrus peel–like

Blends Well With: Citronella, clary sage, lavandin, lavender, neroli, rosemary

Perfumery Note: Top

Aromatherapy Classification: Energizing

Ayurvedic Classification: Vata or air
Flash Point: 115° F.
Safety: Nontoxic, very mild irritant, nonphototoxic, nonsensitizing
Storage: Refrigerate
Aromatherapy Applications: Energizing, uplifting
Skin Care Applications: Blemished skin, oily skin, waterlogged skin
AVEDA Products: Elixir; Exfoliant; Key Element—2 water nature (Aroma), 7 air water nature, 25 infinity nature (Aroma); Purifying Mist—Insightful, Nurturing; Valencia Aroma Diffuser Oil; and other products

MANDARIN OIL

Source: Mandarin
Description: Brownish-orange, clear liquid
Part Used: Fruit peels
Preparation Method: Expression
Olfactory Description: Citrus; strong, deep, sweet fresh citrus, with hint of earthy, heavy neroli-type note
Blends Well With: Basil, bergamot, chamomile, clary sage, frankincense, geranium, grapefruit, lavender, lemon, lime, neroli, orange, rose
Perfumery Note: Top-middle
Aromatherapy Classification: Calming
Ayurvedic Classification: Vata or air
Flash Point: 120° F.
Safety: Nontoxic, nonirritant, nonphototoxic, nonsensitizing
Storage: Refrigerate
Aromatherapy Applications: Calming, tonifying
Skin Care Applications: Blemished skin, oily skin, waterlogged skin
AVEDA Products: All Chakra V products; Indigenous Pure-fume— Gaia Absolute; Key Element—1 earth nature (Aroma), 13 earth nature (Aroma); and other products

MELISSA OIL

Source: Lemon balm
Description: Clear pale yellow, oily liquid
Parts Used: Aerial parts
Preparation Method: Steam distillation
Olfactory Description: Citrus; fresh, citrusy, reminiscent of citronella
Blends Well With: Basil, bay, chamomile, frankincense, geranium, ginger, guaiacwood, jasmine, juniper, lavender, marjoram, neroli, rose, rosemary, violet, ylang-ylang
Perfumery Note: Top-middle
Aromatherapy Classification: Calming
Ayurvedic Classification: Pitta or fire
Flash Point: >200° F.
Safety: Nontoxic, nonirritant, nonphototoxic, nonsensitizing
Storage: Store in a tightly sealed container away from heat and light
Aromatherapy Application: Soothing agent
Skin Care Application: Inflamed skin
AVEDA Products: Relax Cleanser, Self-Timing Perm, and other products

MARJORAM OIL

Source: Sweet marjoram
Description: Clear pale yellow, oily liquid
Part Used: Flowering tops
Preparation Method: Steam distillation
Olfactory Description: Camphoraceous; clean soft character
Aromatherapy Classification: Calming
Ayurvedic Classification: Vata or air
Flash Point: 126° F.
Safety: Nontoxic, nonirritant, nonsensitizing, nonphototoxic, should not be used by pregnant women
Storage: Store in cool, dry area in closed containers; do not expose to high temperatures.
Skin Care Application: Not used
AVEDA Products: Active Composition, Adaptive Cleansing Base, Shampure, and other products

MYRRH OIL

Source: Myrrh
Description: Amber to dark greenish brown, clear mobile aromatic oily liquid
Part Used: Resin
Preparation Method: Steam distillation
Olfactory Description: Balsamic
Aromatherapy Classification: Calming
Ayurvedic Classification: Kapha or earth/water
Flash Point: 110° F.
Safety: Mildly toxic, nonirritant, nonsensitizing, nonphototoxic
Storage: Store in tightly sealed container
Aromatherapy Applications: Insect repellent, emollient
Skin Care Application: Mature skin
AVEDA Products: All Chakra I products, all Chakra V products, and other products

MYRTLE OIL

Source: Myrtle
Description: Clear yellow to green liquid
Part Used: Flowering tops
Preparation Method: Steam distillation
Olfactory Description: Camphoraceous; fresh, slightly sweet, and penetrating; camphoraceous and peppery green aroma, like bay
Blends Well With: Bergamot, cardamom, coriander, dill, lavender, lemon, lemongrass, rosemary, rosewood, spearmint, tea tree, thyme
Perfumery Note: Top-middle
Aromatherapy Classification: Energizing
Ayurvedic Classification: Kapha or earth/water
Flash Point: >95° F.
Safety: Highly toxic orally; undiluted oil may be irritating to eyes, skin, and mucous membranes; prolonged or repeated contact may cause allergenic dermatitis
Storage: Refrigerate
Aromatherapy Applications: Tonifying, stimulating

MYRTLE OIL *(continued)*

Skin Care Applications: Blemished skin, oily skin

AVEDA Products: Skin Firming/Toning Agent and other products

NEROLI OIL

Source: Bitter orange

Description: Clear amber-yellow, clear mobile oily liquid

Part Used: Flowers

Preparation Method: Steam distillation

Olfactory Description: Citrus; sweet bitter floral, with citrus undernote

Blends Well With: Citrus oils, jasmine, rose, ylang-ylang

Perfumery Note: Top-middle

Aromatherapy Classification: Energizing

Ayurvedic Classification: Pitta or fire

Flash Point: 122° F.

Safety: Nonirritating, nonsensitizing, nonphototoxic

Storage: Refrigerate

Aromatherapy Applications: Stimulating, balancing, uplifting, antimicrobial (preserving)

Skin Care Applications: All types, blemished skin, mature skin, normal/combination skin, sensitive skin

AVEDA Products: Key Element 29 full spectrum (Aroma), Lavandou Aroma Diffuser Oil, Lavandou Aroma Mist, Lavandou Candle, Miraculous Beauty Replenisher, and other products

NUTMEG OIL

Source: Nutmeg

Description: Pale yellow, clear aromatic oily liquid

Part Used: Fruits

Preparation Method: Steam distillation

Olfactory Description: Spice note; smooth sweet spicy, with musky undernote similar to juniper berries

Blends Well With: Balsam peru, bay leaf, clary sage, coriander, geranium,

lavandin, lime, mandarin, oakmoss, orange, petitgrain, rosemary

Perfumery Note: Top-middle-base

Aromatherapy Classification: Energizing

Ayurvedic Classification: Kapha or earth/water

Flash Point: 140° F.

Safety: Use ½ recommended dilution or less; slight oral toxicity

Storage: Refrigerate

Aromatherapy Applications: Energizing, stimulating, warming

Skin Care Application: Not used

AVEDA Products: Indigenous Pure-fume—Mizan Absolute, Mizan Spirit; Key Element—1 earth nature (Aroma), 3 fire nature (Aroma); and other products

OLIBANUM OIL

Source: Olibanum

Description: Pale yellow, clear aromatic oily liquid

Part Used: Resin

Preparation Method: Steam distillation

Olfactory Description: Balsamic; balsamic spicy, penetrating camphoraceous, with sweet undernote

Blends Well With: Basil, black pepper, galbanum, geranium, grapefruit, lavender, melissa, orange, patchouli, pine, sandalwood

Perfumery Note: Top-middle-base

Aromatherapy Classification: Energizing

Ayurvedic Classification: Kapha or earth/water

Flash Point: 95° F.

Safety: Flammable; nonirritating, nonsensitizing, nonphototoxic

Storage: Room temperature

Aromatherapy Applications: Stimulating, tonifying, grounding

Skin Care Applications: Mature skin, normal/combination skin, oily skin

AVEDA Products: All Chakra II products; Indigenous Pure-fume—Mizan Absolute, Mizan Spirit; Singular Notes—Olibanum; and other products

ORANGE OIL

Source: Bitter orange

Description: Intense yellow to golden yellow, clear oily liquid

Part Used: Fruit peels

Preparation Method: Expression

Olfactory Description: Citrus; sweet citrus orange peel–like

Blends Well With: All citrus oils, neroli, orange flower, petitgrain

Perfumery Note: Top

Aromatherapy Classification: Calming

Ayurvedic Classifications: Kapha or earth/water, pitta or fire, vata or air

Flash Point: 115° F.

Safety: Nontoxic, nonirritant, nonphototoxic, nonsensitizing

Storage: Store in full sealed containers in cool, dry place away from sources of ignition heat or direct sunlight; follow good industrial and hygenic practices

Aromatherapy Application: Astringent

Skin Care Application: Skin conditioning

AVEDA Products: Key Element—1 earth nature (Aroma), 5 infinity nature, 6 water air nature, 9 water air fire nature; Shampure; and other products

OTTO ROSE

Source: Rose, damask

Description: Pale yellow to greenish yellow, clear aromatic liquid

Part Used: Flowers

Preparation Method: Steam distillation

Olfactory Description: Woody; intensly sweet, but a touch of light, fresh floral note

Blends Well With: Virtually all florals, especially jasmine

Perfumery Note: Top-middle

Aromatherapy Classification: Calming

Ayurvedic Classification: Pitta or fire

Flash Point: 185° F.

Safety: Slight skin irritant

Storage: Refrigerate

Aromatherapy Applications: Cooling, balancing, calming, tonifying

Skin Care Applications: Dry skin, mature skin, normal/combination skin, sensitive skin

AVEDA Products: Indigenous Pure-fume—Hana Absolute, Hana Spirit; Key Element 9 water air fire nature; Styling Curessence; and other products

PALMAROSA OIL

Source: Palmarosa

Description: Light yellow to yellow, clear liquid

Parts Used: Aerial parts

Preparation Method: Steam distillation

Olfactory Description: Floral; sweet, floral-rosy aroma and dry grasslike undertones

Blends Well With: Amyris, bois de rose, cananga, geranium, guaicawood, oakmoss

Perfumery Note: Top-middle-base

Aromatherapy Classification: Calming

Ayurvedic Classification: Kapha or earth/water

Flash Point: 65° F.

Safety: Low irritation potential, nonsensitizing, nonphototoxic

Storage: Room temperature

Aromatherapy Applications: Soothing, calming

Skin Care Applications: Blemished skin, dry skin, normal/combination skin

AVEDA Products: Hydrating Lotion, Purescriptions Elixir Remedy, Refreshing Bath Bar, Smoothing Body Polish, Soothing Aqua Therapy, and other products

PATCHOULI OIL

Source: Patchouli

Description: Light amber to deep straw yellow, clear oily liquid

Part Used: Leaves

Preparation Method: Steam distillation

Olfactory Description: Woody; deep woody with a hint of camphoraceous top note and musty earthy chocolatelike sweet undernote; freshly distilled oils may have a greenish look and harsh note; aging the oil is of the utmost importance; an oil several years old will possess a much finer and fuller aroma than a freshly distilled oil; the aroma imparts strength and is full-bodied with alluring notes of lasting quality when the oil has been properly aged

Blends Well With: Bergamot, cedarwood, clary sage, clove, geranium, labdanum, lavender, myrrh, neroli, oakmoss, rose, sandalwood, vetiver

Perfumery Note: Top-middle-base

Aromatherapy Classification: Calming

Ayurvedic Classification: Vata or air

Flash Point: 200° F.

Safety: Nontoxic, nonirritant, nonphototoxic, nonsensitizing

Storage: Store in fully sealed containers in cool, dry place away from sources of ignition heat or direct sunlight; follow good industrial and hygenic practices

Aromatherapy Applications: Antiseptic, astringent, aphrodisiac, perfume

Skin Care Applications: Blemished skin, oily skin

AVEDA Products: Adaptive Bath Essence Base; After Shave Balm; Curessence; Indigenous Pure-fume—Amazonia Absolute, Amazonia Spirit; Key Element—2 water nature (Aroma), 6 water air nature, 15 water nature (Aroma), 29 full spectrum (Aroma); Styling Curessence; and other products

PEPPERMINT OIL

Source: Mint, peppermint

Description: Colorless to pale yellow, clear thin liquid

Parts Used: Aerial parts

Preparation Method: Steam distillation

Olfactory Description: Minty; strong, minty-herbaceous note with balsamic-sweet undertones, truly reminiscent of the plant; the aroma of peppermint becomes increasingly mellow and beautiful with time; newly distilled oil generally has a weedy note, which decreases noticeably after three months of storage

Blends Well With: Bergamot, cornmint, geranium oil, lavender oil, marjoram, rosemary, sandalwood

Perfumery Note: Top-middle

Aromatherapy Classification: Energizing

Ayurvedic Classifications: Kapha or earth/water, vata or air

Flash Point: 160° F.

Safety: Nonflammable

Storage: Room temperature

Aromatherapy Applications: Stimulant, decongestant

Skin Care Applications: Blemished skin, dry skin

AVEDA Products: Active Composition; Key Element—1 earth nature (Aroma), 12 earth nature (Aroma); Rosemary/Mint Equalizer; Singular Notes—Peppermint; and other products

PETITGRAIN OIL

Source: Bitter orange

Description: Yellow to brownish yellow, clear mobile liquid

Parts Used: Leaves and stems

Preparation Method: Steam distillation

Olfactory Description: Citrus

Aromatherapy Classification: Calming

Ayurvedic Classification: Pitta or fire

Flash Point: 152° F.

Safety: Nontoxic, very mild irritant, nonphototoxic, nonsensitizing

Storage: Store in a cool area away from heat and flames

Aromatherapy Applications: Balancing the nervous system—inhaled for nervous exhaustion, fatigue, or stress

Skin Care Application: Blemished skin

PETITGRAIN OIL (*continued*)

AVEDA Products: Chi Body Compound, Chi Cleanser, Sunsource, and other products

PIMENTO BERRY OIL

Source: Pimento
Description: Clear pale yellow, oily liquid
Part Used: Fruits
Preparation Method: Steam distillation
Olfactory Description: Spice note; warm sweet spicy, reminiscent of clove
Blends Well With: Geranium, ginger, labdanum, lavender, opoponax, orris, patchouli, ylang-ylang
Perfumery Note: Top-middle
Aromatherapy Classification: Energizing
Ayurvedic Classification: Kapha or earth/water
Flash Point: >200° F.
Safety: Use ½ recommended dilution or less; can cause skin irritation; orally moderately toxic
Storage: Store in tight full containers in a cool, dry place away from light
Aromatherapy Applications: Energizing, stimulating
Skin Care Application: Not used
AVEDA Products: Pimento Berry Pure Essence, Unisex Soap Holiday '98, and other products

ROSE ABSOLUTE

Source: Rose, damask
Description: Orange-yellow, oily mobile liquid
Part Used: Flowers
Preparation Method: Solvent extraction
Olfactory Description: Floral; deep floral, woody sweet, but spicy honeylike undernote
Perfumery Note: Top-middle
Aromatherapy Classification: Calming
Ayurvedic Classification: Pitta or fire
Flash Point: >200° F.
Safety: Nontoxic, very mild irritant, nonphototoxic, nonsensitizing

Storage: Store in a cool area away from heat and flames
Aromatherapy Applications: Perfume, skin conditioner, aphrodisiac
Skin Care Applications: Dry skin, mature skin, normal/combination skin, sensitive skin
AVEDA Products: Purescriptions Dry Remedy and other products

ROSEMARY OIL

Source: Rosemary
Description: Water white to pale yellow, clear thin liquid
Part Used: Flowering tops
Preparation Method: Steam distillation
Olfactory Description: Camphoraceous; fresh, strong herbaceous, similar to lavender note, with pronounced camphoraceous medicinal note and woody-balsamic undernote
Blends Well With: Basil, cedarwood, cinnamon, citronella, elemi, labdanum, lavandin, lavender, olibanum, oregano, peppermint, petitgrain, pine, thyme
Perfumery Note: Top-middle
Aromatherapy Classification: Energizing
Ayurvedic Classifications: Kapha or earth/water, vata or air
Flash Point: 113° F.
Safety: Nontoxic, nonirritant, nonphototoxic, nonsensitizing
Storage: Store in a cool area away from heat and flames
Aromatherapy Applications: Muscle relaxant, soothing agent
Skin Care Applications: Blemished skin, oily skin. Note: Skin conditioning
AVEDA Products: Hydrating Lotion, Purifying Creme Cleanser, Purifying Gel Cleanser, and other products

SAGE OIL

Source: Sage, dalmatian
Description: Clear colorless to yellow liquid

Part Used: Leaves
Preparation Method: Steam distillation
Olfactory Description: Camphoraceous; refreshing camphoraceous, with spicy warm undertone
Blends Well With: Bois de rose, citrus, lavandin, rosemary
Perfumery Note: Top-middle
Aromatherapy Classification: Energizing
Ayurvedic Classification: Vata or air
Flash Point: 130°
Safety: Should be avoided by pregnant women, small children, and those with epilepsy
Storage: Refrigerate
Aromatherapy Applications: Calming, grounding, antimicrobial (preserving)
Skin Care Applications: Blemished skin, mature skin, oily skin
AVEDA Products: Energizing Composition and other products

SANDALWOOD OIL

Source: Sandalwood, Indian
Description: Pale yellow to amber yellow, clear liquid
Part Used: Wood
Preparation Method: Steam distillation
Olfactory Description: Woody; sweet-woody balsamic, with rich, warm, earthy undernote
Blends Well With: Benzoin, bergamot, black pepper, cassie, clove, costus, geranium, jasmine, labdanum, lavender, mimosa, myrrh, oakmoss, patchouli, rose, rosewood, tuberose, vetiver, violet
Perfumery Note: Middle-base
Aromatherapy Classification: Calming
Ayurvedic Classification: Pitta or fire
Flash Point: >200° F.
Safety: OK; low potential for irritation and sensitivity
Storage: Room temperature
Aromatherapy Applications: Emollient, soothing agent, astringent, insect repellent
Skin Care Applications: Blemished skin, dry skin, oily skin, sensitive skin. Note: Skin conditioning

AVEDA Products: Calming Composition; all Chakra I products; all Chakra II products; all Chakra VI products; Key Element—2 water nature (Aroma), 9 water air fire nature, 21 air nature (Aroma); Lavandou Aroma Diffuser Oil; Lavandou Aroma Mist; Love; Miraculous Beauty Replenisher; Purescriptions Dry Remedy; Singular Notes—Sandalwood; and other products

SPEARMINT OIL

Source: Mint, spearmint
Description: Colorless to greenish yellow, clear mobile oily liquid
Part Used: Flowering tops
Preparation Method: Steam distillation
Olfactory Description: Minty; a warm, sweet fresh green-minty, slightly herbaceous note
Blends Well With: Bergamot, jasmine, lavender, sandalwood
Perfumery Note: Top-middle
Aromatherapy Classification: Calming
Ayurvedic Classification: Kapha or earth/water
Flash Point: 137° F.
Safety: Use ½ recommended dilution or less; nonirritating, nonsensitizing, nonphototoxic
Storage: Refrigerate
Aromatherapy Applications: Calming
Skin Care Applications: Blemished skin, oily skin
AVEDA Products: Shave Emollient and other products

TEA TREE OIL

Source: Tea tree
Description: Clear pale to light yellow, mobile oily liquid

Parts Used: Leaves and stems
Preparation Method: Steam distillation
Olfactory Description: Aromatic; fresh medicinal camphoraceous, hint of citrus and piney undernote
Blends Well With: Cananga, clary sage, clove, geranium, lavandin, lavender, marjoram, nutmeg, oakmoss, pine, rosemary
Perfumery Note: Top-middle-base
Aromatherapy Classification: Energizing
Ayurvedic Classification: Kapha or earth/water
Flash Point: 130° F.
Safety: Slight oral toxicity
Storage: Refrigerate
Aromatherapy Applications: Antimicrobial, stimulant, decongestant
Skin Care Applications: Blemished skin, oily skin
AVEDA Products: Singular Notes—Tea Tree—and other products

VANILLA ABSOLUTE

Source: Vanilla
Description: Dark brown or amber, clear mobile aromatic liquid
Part Used: Seeds
Preparation Method: Solvent extraction
Olfactory Description: Spice note; very typical sweet, warm, with balsamic undertone
Blends Well With: Benzoin, opopanax, sandalwood, vetiver
Perfumery Note: Top-middle-base
Aromatherapy Classification: Calming
Ayurvedic Classification: Kapha or earth/water
Flash Point: >200° F.
Safety: Nontoxic, nonirritant, nonphototoxic, nonsensitizing
Storage: Refrigerate
Aromatherapy Applications: Emollient, aphrodisiac

Skin Care Application: Not used
AVEDA Products: Adaptive Cleansing Base; all Chakra VI products; Confixor; Confixor—Low VOC; Key Element—3 fire nature (Aroma), 15 water nature (Aroma); Madagascar Aroma Diffuser Oil; Madagascar Aroma Mist; Shampure; Singular Notes—Vanilla; Total Body Cleanser; and other products

VETIVER OIL

Source: Vetiver
Description: Clear amber liquid
Part Used: Roots
Preparation Method: Steam distillation
Olfactory Description: Woody; earthy-woody, with earthy weedy wet impression and sweet undertones
Blends Well With: Cassie, clary sage, jasmine, lavender, mimosa, oakmoss, opopanax, patchouli, sandalwood, ylang-ylang
Perfumery Note: Middle-base
Aromatherapy Classifications: Calming
Ayurvedic Classifications: Testing is in process.
Flash Point: 194° F.
Safety: OK; nonirritating, nonsensitizing; low toxicity potential
Storage: Room temperature
Aromatherapy Applications: Balancing, grounding
Skin Care Applications: Inflamed skin, mature skin, sensitive skin. Note: Toxic—use ½ recommended dilution
AVEDA Products: All Chakra II products, all Chakra VI products, Key Element 3 fire nature (Aroma), and other products

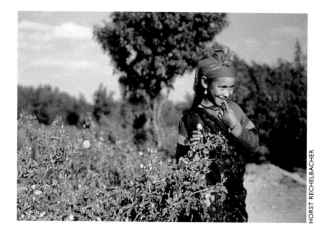

Resources

Following are some books, journals, and organizations to which I refer you for further information on health, organics, environmentalism, and activism. I encourage you to take your rituals beyond the microcosmos of the individual self and to contribute to positive change in the world around you.

BOOKS

Brown, Lester R., Christopher Flavin, Hilary French. *State of the World: A Worldwatch Report on Progress Toward a Sustainable Society.* New York: W.W. Norton and Co., 1998.

Colborn, Theo, Dianne Dumanoski, and John Peterson Myers. *Our Stolen Future: Are We Threatening Our Fertility, Intelligence, and Survival?—A Scientific Detective Story.* New York: Plume, 1997.

Gips, Teri. *Breaking the Pesticide Habit.* Minneapolis: International Alliance, 1988.

Globally and Locally: Seeking a Middle Path to Sustainable Development, ed. Alan McQuillan and Ashley Preston. University Press of America, 1998.

Hawken, Paul. *Ecology of Commerce: A Declaration of Sustainability.* New York: HarperBusiness, 1994.

Logan, Karen Noonan. *Clean House, Clean Planet: Manual to Free Your Home of 14 Common Hazard Household Products.* New York: Pocket Books, 1997.

Martin, Alice T. *Students Shopping for a Better World.* New York: Council on Economic Priorities, 1993.

National Green Pages. Washington, D.C.: Co-op America, annual, (800) 58-GREEN. www.coopamerica.org

Robbins, John. *Diet for a New America: How Your Food Choices Affect Your Health, Happiness and the Future of Life on Earth.* Tiburon, Calif.: H. J. Kramer, 1998.

World Resources Institute and Joyce Vedral. *World Resources: A Guide to the Global Environment*. New York: Oxford University Press, 1998.

JOURNALS

Business Ethics, P.O. Box 8439, Minneapolis, MN 55408. BizEthics@aol.com

Consumer Currents, 24 Highbury Crescent, London N5 1RX, United Kingdom. http://www.consumersinternational.org

Co-op America Quarterly, Co-op America, Inc., 2100 M Street, NW, Ste. 310, Washington, DC 20063.

Ecoforum, Environmental Liaison Center International, Nairobi, Kenya.

Green Business Letter, Tilden Press, Inc., 1519 Connecticut Avenue NW, Washington, DC 20036, (202) 332-1700. gbl@enm.com, www.enn.com/gbl

Mother Jones Magazine, 731 Market Street, #600, San Francisco, CA 94103, (415) 665-6637. www.mother.jones.com

World Watch Magazine, World Watch Institute, 1776 Massachusetts Ave. NW, Washington, DC 20063.

ORGANIZATIONS

Alliance for Sustainability, 1701 University Ave. SE, Minneapolis, MN 55414, (612) 331-1099. tgips@mtn.org, www.mtn.org/iasa

Business for Social Responsibility, 609 Mission St., 2nd floor, San Francisco, CA 94105.

Center for Science in the Public Interest (CSPI), 1501 16th St. NW, Washington, DC 20036, (202) 332-9110.

Consumer Policy Institute, c/o Consumer Union, 256 Washington St., Mt. Vernon, NY 10553, (914) 667-9400.

Co-op America, 1612 K Street NW, #600, Washington, DC 20006, (800) 58-GREEN. www.coopamerica.org

Council on Economic Priorities (CEP), 30 Irving Place, New York, NY 10003, (212) 420-1133. cep@echonyc.com

Ecological Agriculture Projects (EAP), Box 225, Macdonald College, Ste. Anne de Bellevue, Quebec H9X1CO.

Foundation on Economic Trends (FET), 1130 17th Street NW, Washington, DC 20036, (202) 466-2823.

Friends of the Earth (FOE), 377 City Road, London, England, or FOE, 530 7th St. SE, Washington, DC 20003, (202) 543-4312.

Fundación Natura, Casilla 253, Quito, Ecuador 249780.

Greenpeace, Greenpeace USA, 1611 Connecticut Ave. NW, Washington, DC 20007, (202) 462-1177.

Institute for Food and Development Policy (Food First), 145 Ninth St., San Francisco, CA 94103, (415) 864-8555.

International Federation of Organic Agriculture Movements (IFOAM), c/o Okozentrum Imsbach, D-6695 Tholey-Theley, Federal Republic of Germany, 0-68-53/51-90.

National Audubon Society, NAS, 645 Pennsylvania Ave., SE, Washington, DC 20003, (202) 547-9009.

National Coalition Against the Misuse of Pesticides (NCAMP), 530 7th St. SE, Washington, DC 20003, (202) 543-5450.

Natural Resource Defense Council (NRDC), 122 E. 42nd St., New York, NY 10168, (212) 949-0049.

Natural Step, International. http://www.naturalstep.org/what/index_intl.html

Natural Step, USA, P.O. Box 20672, San Francisco, CA 94129, (415) 561-3344. tns@naturalstep.org

New England Organic Farmer's Association (NEOFA), 43 State St., Montpelier, VT 05602, (802) 454-8550.

Organic Food Production Association of North America (OFPANA), P.O. Box 31, Belchertown, MA 01007.

Permaculture Institute, P.O. Box 96, Stanley, Tasmania, Australia 7331, (004) 581142.

Pesticide Action Network, 49 Power St., 5th Floor, San Francisco, CA 94102.

Pesticide Action Network, North American Regional Center (formerly Pesticide Education and Action Project PEAP) (PAN NARC), 965 Mission St., Se. 514, San Francisco, CA 94103, (415) 981-1771.

Rocky Mountain Institute, 1739 Snowmass Creek Rd., Snowmass, CO 81654, (970) 927-3851. www.rmi.org

Sierra Club International, 29 Sawer Ave., Medford, MA 02155.

U.S. Environment Protection Agency (U.S. EPA), Washington, DC 20460, (703) 557-5017.

United Farm Workers, AFL-CIO (UFW), P.O. Box 62, Keene, CA 93531, (805) 822-5571.

United Nations Environment Programme (UNEP), P.O. Box 30552, Nairobi, Kenya.

Working Weekends on Organic Farms (WWOOF), 19 Bradford Rd., Lewes, E. Sussex, England, BN71RB.

World Resources Institute (WRI), 1735 New York Ave. NW, Washington, DC 20006, (202) 638-6300.

RETAIL STORES/CATALOGS

Harmony, Seventh Generation Catalog, 360 Interlocken Blvd., Suite 300, Broomfield, CO 80021, (800) 869-3446.

Clean House, Clean Planet, 23852 Pacific Coast Hwy., #200, Malibu, CA 90265, (818) 880-5144. www.cleanhouse.com

Real Goods Trading Company, 555 Leslie Street, Ukiah, CA 95482, (707) 468-9292.

Index

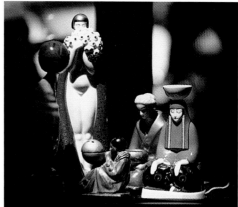

HORST RECHELBACHER